W9-AMR-547

LIQUID HERBAL DROPS IN EVERYDAY USE

4TH EDITION

DANIEL GAGNON
medical herbalist

Botanical Research and Education Institute, Inc.

....

Please note!

This book is designed to provide you with herbal care options. Keep in mind that the herbs listed in this book are for prevention and for problems that do not require major medical intervention. This book is not intended to replace the expertise of a primary care practitioner. If the complaint you are treating is not getting better, or if it is getting worse, consult a doctor. The publisher, the author, and the editors do not assume any responsibility for any injury and/or damage to persons or property arising out of or related to any use of the material contained in this book. The reader is advised to check the appropriate literature and the product information currently provided by the manufacturer of each therapeutic substance to verify dosages, the method and duration of administration, contraindications or side effects.

AUTHOR: Daniel Gagnon
EDITOR: Jerilynn Blum and Nicole Osterhaus
EDITORIAL ASSISTANT: Christa Weidner-Sandoval
PUBLISHING CONSULTANT: Kristie Peterson
EDITORIAL CONSULTANTS: Melissa Stofan Berry,
    Kelly McDowell, Jamie Reagan
GRAPHIC DESIGN: John Cole
BOOK & COVER ILLUSTRATIONS: Angela Werneke
    (© 1995 Angela Werneke)
COVER PHOTOGRAPHY: Don Gregg, Hawthorne Studios

Copyright ©2000, 1996 by Daniel J. Gagnon

First Edition 1993	50,000 copies sold
Second Edition 1996	20,000 copies sold
Third Edition 1997	35,000 copies sold
Fourth Edition 2000	15,000 copies printed

ALL RIGHTS RESERVED. No part of this book may be reproduced in any form or by any electronic or mechanical means, including information storage and retrieval systems, without permission in writing from the author except by a reviewer who may quote brief passages in a review.

Publisher: Botanical Research & Education Institute, Inc.
    2442 Cerrillos Road, Suite 296
    Santa Fe, NM 87505

♻ Post consumer recycled paper

About Daniel Gagnon

Daniel has been a practicing herbalist since 1976. Born in French Canada, he relocated to Santa Fe, New Mexico in 1979. There he furthered his studies in medical herbalism, pharmacognosy and related subjects at the Santa Fe College of Natural Medicine, the College of Santa Fe and the College of Pharmacy at the University of New Mexico.

His passion for helping others was born out of his own childhood health problems. His experience with conventional medical treatment of eczema, asthma and allergies motivated him to seek gentler, more soothing healing modalities, which ultimately put him on the path to becoming an herbalist. His goal is to educate both the public and the medical profession about the practical, healing applications of herbal medicine.

Health care professionals such as medical doctors, naturopaths, chiropractors and acupuncturists frequently call upon Daniel as an herbal consultant. He is the co-author of *Breathe Free*, a nutritional and herbal care book for the respiratory system; and the author of *Healing Herbs for the Nervous System*. He regularly teaches seminars and classes on herbal therapeutics, both nationally and internationally. He is senior professor of Materia Medica at the North American College of Botanical Medicine. The College, located in Albuquerque, New Mexico, offers a three-year herbalist training program.

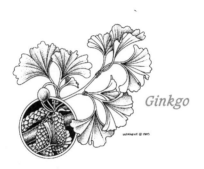

Ginkgo

Table of Contents

Author's Introduction:
About This Book

September 2000, Fourth Edition

Dear Herbal Enthusiast,

My goal in writing *Liquid Herbal Drops in Everyday Use*—whether you are just beginning to learn about herbs or whether you are already knowledgeable— is to provide you with the best, most practical, easy-reference guide to herbal medicine in the marketplace today. In fact, many consumers have called *Liquid Herbal Drops in Everyday Use* a "gold mine" of herbal information. There are many books that generally detail "which herbs are good for what." What this book does differently is to help you focus, in practical and specific terms, on which herbs to take at what times and how best to take them. It also warns you about contraindications, possible side effects and/or warnings.

It has been inspiring to receive such positive feedback on the first, second and third editions of this book. I never expected that over 100,000 copies would be sold in less than seven years!

Thank you to all the readers who wrote to say how useful the book was to them. I also appreciate those who wrote to make specific suggestions on how to improve this book.

In this fourth edition, we have incorporated many new features that were suggested by readers, as well as friends, fellow retailers and health professionals. We have redone the Questions and Answers section to incorporate all the

Calendula

new information that has made its way into herbal literature. The **Herbal Directory** grows to include 22 new single extracts and formulas. The **Health Condition Index** has been expanded and simplified; it is easier to find which herb may offer the best results in over 370 different health conditions. Most importantly, we have worked diligently to keep the price of this book low so that more people can benefit from this valuable information.

The formulas listed in this book are ones that I have put together over the past ten years. I recommend them in my practice as a Medical Herbalist and also in my role as a consultant to professional healthcare practitioners.

All the formulas listed have been tested and improved upon as a result of ongoing scientific testing and/or client feedback; and all have proven to be safe and effective. These formulas are available at natural food markets, herb stores and natural pharmacies throughout the United States and Canada.

I welcome any of your suggestions or comments on how this book can be improved for the next edition. I also want to hear about your ideas on what additional herbs should be included next time.

I thank all the people that have helped me create this book—be it employees, professionals, retailers, and consumers.

I hope you enjoy reading this book. May it enlighten you with helpful insights and point the way in your quest for health.

Herbally Yours,

Daniel Gagnon

Chapter 1:

The Ten Elements of Good Health

Remember, you are a physical, mental, emotional and spiritual ecosystem....

It is important to understand that good physical health does not exist independently of our thoughts, feelings, beliefs and the lifestyle decisions we make. We each exist in a personal and collective ecosystem where both internal processes and external factors affect our bodies. No system of health care, herbal or otherwise, can "cure" a physical condition that exists within an ecosystem that is out of balance.

Personal choice is the key to maintaining the health of our ecosystems. We are the sum of the choices that we make every day. Moment to moment, we choose what to think, what to eat and drink, who to be with, what to talk about, when to exercise, how much sleep to get, and so forth. All of these choices may seem insignificant when we make them one by one, but, added together, they have a tremendous impact on our bodies. For example, going to a fast food place occasionally does not have major health consequences. But when fast foods are our main food supply, two things happen simultaneously; our bodies become overloaded with fats, sodium and free radicals as well as becoming starved for fiber, vitamins and minerals. Over a period of time, this type of diet leads to degenerative diseases. It may take years, but it will happen. The bottom line is that each choice we make either adds up to "health enhancing" or "health depleting".

Maintaining our ecosystem is a dynamic process that is a little bit like being on a seesaw. As we move away from our center, our energy is sapped so that we are more subject to extreme highs and lows. Conversely, the closer we move toward our pivot point of balance, the less energy we need to expend to stay healthy. The surplus energy that is created by being more balanced can then be used for doing things in our lives that give us joy, happiness and contentment. Our bodies can also utilize this energy for repairing themselves and maintaining optimal health.

Actually, optimal health is incredibly simple to attain and maintain if one is personally attentive to the ten elements of health. By far, most of us get sick because we neglect the basics. On top of that, our society has taught us to be overly dependent on experts, pills, and surgery to maintain and take charge of our health. Many doctors also perpetuate this dependency by not being alert to these ten essential elements of health.

The good news is that you don't need detailed scientific or medical knowledge to take charge of your health. If you wish to optimize your health and increase your resilience, or if you are confronted with a health problem, I suggest examining how balanced you are in the following ten areas. What choices are you making in these ten areas? Balancing these ten elements on a daily basis leads to good health and helps keep you there.

1. CHOICE Are you taking personal responsibility for your life?

A critical step in the self-creation of a healthy body and a healthy life involves taking daily responsibility for your actions. Taking personal responsibility for your well being is such an important element that, by itself, it accounts for 40% of healing. At any given moment, we have choice. Exercising choice in healthy ways is the key that unlocks the door to integrating and balancing all of the other elements of healthy living discussed in the following pages.

2. EXERCISE Are you exercising regularly?

Exercise at least five times a week for one-half to three-quarters of an hour. One of the best forms of exercise is walking because it is low impact, cardiovascular, and inexpensive! The importance of exercise cannot be underestimated, as it is a critical element in maintaining your entire ecosystem.

Damiana

9

3. REST Are you getting enough rest and sleep?
Set aside some time every day just to do nothing except relax and breathe, even if it is only for 15 minutes. Place a priority on getting enough restful sleep. Sleep time before midnight is the most beneficial. Taking naps during the day is also recommended.

4. NUTRITION Is your diet fully supporting your body?
Eat whole foods and organic foods. Eat a variety of whole grains, vegetables and fruits. Include at least one portion a day of any of the following green leafy vegetables: Swiss and red chard, kale, collards, Brussels sprouts, parsley, mustard greens, turnip greens, chicory greens, dandelion or beet greens, spinach, cabbage, watercress, purslane, okra, broccoli, or any sprouts, including alfalfa, sunflower and soybean. Vitamins and minerals are helpful in supplementing your diet, even if you are eating organic foods. Take a full spectrum vitamin/mineral supplement every day. Drink half an ounce of water per pound of body weight a day to stay fully hydrated (about eight eight-ounce glasses a day). Don't forget to take your herbs.

5. NATURE Do you spend enough time outdoors?
Nothing can replace being in nature when it comes down to balancing yourself. Devoting time daily to getting fresh air and sun is critical to the overall health of your personal ecosystem. When you are out walking (see element 2), consider doing so in a natural place, removed from traffic, power lines and noise.

6. CREATIVITY Do you have some sort of creative outlet that keeps you active physically and mentally?
A creative outlet can range from work to that hobby you never seem to have time for. Working in moderation in a domain that you like is nurturing, self-affirming and rewarding. Staying active and in contact with the rest of the world is integral to good health.

7. EMOTIONAL BALANCE Are you emotionally healthy?
Do you have anger, fear or grief that keeps you out of balance? There is nothing wrong with having feelings. They give us valuable information about what we may

need to change in our lives to be happy. Emotional imbalance becomes an issue when feelings are allowed to either create internal harm to the self or external harm to others. If either of these extremes is true for you, take measures to identify and balance your emotional patterns. Choose to cultivate joy, love and a sense of humor to nourish your ecosystem.

8. GOALS Are you mentally stimulated?

To thrive, everyone should have something—whether it's doing volunteer work, spearheading a project, or working toward a goal—that demands brain activity. We all need direction and a sense of purpose in life. Goals give meaning to our lives.

9. MUTUAL SUPPORT Are you giving and receiving love in your life?

Having a loving and accepting support system is critical to healing and staying healthy. Humans, by their very nature, are dependent upon relationship. Giving and getting support and love from your family, friends, or support group is essential to good health.

10. FAITH Do you regularly communicate with your Higher Self or your Higher Power?

A wise soul once said that we must feel connected to a higher power to feel balanced and fulfilled in life. In keeping with your personal belief system, make time daily for this aspect of yourself or for spiritual guidance to help you in your daily life.

Herbs truly have the ability to assist you in making significant shifts in both chronic and acute physical conditions. The success of herbs in supporting your ecosystem, however, is dependent upon how balanced you are in these ten essential areas. Is there anything missing in your life? What does your personal ecosystem need? Remember that the choices you make daily give you the power to shape your life!

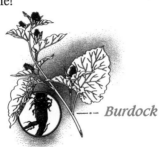

Burdock

11

Chapter 2:

Understanding Herbal Medicine

Q: What is herbal medicine and who uses it?
Herbal medicine, sometimes called botanical medicine or phytotherapy, is the use of herbs for health purposes. Mankind has used herbs for millenniums and thousands of herbs are recognized worldwide for their health benefits. According to the World Health Organization, 80% of the world's population still depends on herbal medicine as a primary form of healing. In the last 25 years, the United States has been going through a major rediscovery of medicinal herbs. During this time, Traditional Chinese Medicine, Ayurvedic Medicine from India, and South American herbs have been assimilated into the American herbal scene.

Q: How does herbal medicine interface with current medical practices?
Herbal medicine for some is a total alternative to conventional allopathic medical treatments. For others, herbal medicine stands alongside conventional medicine as another choice, depending on the health issue at hand. Allopathy is defined as curing an illness or disease by inducing an opposite action in the body. Herbal medicine, on the other hand, supports the body itself to shift.

Overall, herbal medicine offers prevention, affordability, and safety. For these reasons many people see herbal medicine as an alternative to drugs or surgery, which are the treatment modalities most often used in allopathic medicine when health problems reach a crisis point. Drugs often have serious side effects and their costs can be prohibitive. In some instances, the drugs that are given to patients are more dangerous than the illnesses they are intended to treat.

The perspective of herbal medicine practitioners is that conventional allopathic medicine is geared for crisis management, whereas herbal medicine is geared more for preventative measures and chronic conditions. In allopathic medicine, the majority of people go to the doctor when their problems have escalated to the point that they require drastic measures, such as drugs or surgery. Oftentimes, in conventional allopathic medicine, the drugs are too strong or the surgery is too drastic for the problem at hand, however these are sometimes the only treatment options provided.

Herbal medicine offers different choices. Herbs generally assist the healing process by helping rebuild and strengthen weak body systems, causing many nagging health problems to disappear. In the field of holistic medicine, herbs are not taken to "cure" disease but instead are used as tools to help rebalance and support the body in its quest for health.

Q: Specifically, what do herbs offer me in the way of health care benefits?

Herbs offer you eight benefits:

1. Simplicity and accessibility: Herbs are readily available in almost every conceivable delivery system, i.e., capsules, tablets, softgels, tea bags, liquid herbal extracts, loose herbs, lozenges and salves. Most forms of herbs are available at local natural products stores and natural pharmacies.

2. Safety: The bottom line is that herbs are safe but you must, as with any medications, heed dosage recommendations and any contraindications, side effects or warnings that are noted. In the few instances where a pre-existing condition may limit the use of herbs, specific contraindications have been noted for those herbs. In some cases, herbs may cause side effects. These have been noted also. Remember that any substance can have a side effect if enough of it is ingested. For example, eating too many prunes may lead one to discover the laxative effect of these fruits.

Oats

3. Tolerance: Most people do well with herbs. Sometimes conventional drugs have adverse side effects that can only be offset by additional drugs. Herbs, on the other hand, rarely cause such a domino effect.

4. Effectiveness: Herbs are effective despite the fact that they cannot be "tested" in the same manner as drugs. Many "experts" may not recognize herbs with gentle actions as having any therapeutic benefit but anybody who has taken a cup of chamomile tea for sleep problems will attest to the fact that you don't need to be hit over the head with a drug-like effect in order to enjoy the benefits of herbs. Part of the reason that the effects of herbs are not as well documented as drugs is that herbs do not contain just one single active constituent. This makes it challenging for scientists to devise experiments to study herbs, but nevertheless, herbs have been shown for centuries to be effective healing agents.

5. Economy: Many herbs offer the same benefits as drugs for a fraction of what drugs cost. For example, Proscar® costs the average man suffering from benign prostatic hypertrophy (swollen prostate) approximately $2.50 a day for treatment. The same problem can be addressed with the herb Saw Palmetto for about 50 cents a day.

6. Empowerment: Herbs allow you, personally, to do something for your health, at the precise time you need to do it.

7. Ecology for your "ecosystem": Herbs are substances that your body can work with. Herbs are not foreign substances. Therefore, they are easily absorbed and assimilated by the body. They elicit a positive response from the body and aid the body to return to a balanced state.

8. Environmental friendliness: When herbs are certified as organically grown or are ethically wildcrafted, their harvesting has little or no negative impact on the planet. The pharmaceutical industry, on the other hand, manufactures drugs using complex and environmentally negative petroleum by-products and other chemicals.

Q: How do herbs differ from drugs in the way they interact with the body?

There is a fundamental difference between how conventional drugs and herbs interact with the body. Conventional drugs work within the body for a limited time period. Herbs train the body for the future.

Antibiotics, often prescribed by conventional medical practitioners, bypass the immune system to kill intruders; therefore, they do not teach the body how to defend itself in the future. Antibiotics also disrupt the ecology of the body and permit other microorganisms to grow and take over the normal flora in the intestines, as well as in other locations in the body. Drugs leave toxic residues that the body must either detoxify or store.

On the other hand, herbs help reeducate the body to heal itself. For example, Echinacea will stimulate your immune system not only to fight a current infection, but also to recognize intruders quicker and to respond more aggressively the next time your body encounters the same "bug". Because herbs leave no hard-to-deal-with residues, the body regains its full balance much more easily. None of the herbs addressed in this book leave behind hard-to-deal-with residues in the body.

Metaphorically, drugs give a man a fish and feed him for a day. Herbs teach a man how to fish so that he can feed himself for a lifetime.

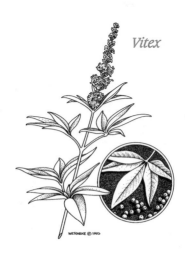

Vitex

WERNEKE © 1995

Chapter 3:

Choosing Which Herbal Products Are Best for You

Q: What forms do herbs come in?
The most popular herbal products in America are capsules, softgels and tablets. Herbal teas, especially in teabags, account for a substantial amount of the herbs consumed in the United States. Herbs in liquid herbal extract form are also a popular way to ingest therapeutic herbal products. Finally, herbs are available in bulk form in some health and natural food stores.

Q: Which form of herbs offers the most therapeutic benefits?
The therapeutic benefits achieved by using herbs depend on a variety of factors. For instance, does the herbal product contain all of the active constituents in ratios found in nature, or have the constituents been altered? Is the herbal product fresh? What is the shelf life of the herbs? Has the herb been processed in such a way as to ensure that it will be effective when you are ready to take the product? Does the product require you to digest the herbs in order to get all of the benefits from these herbs? Is it convenient to take? Is it affordable? Does the product address the problem that you are trying to solve? Of all the available forms of herbs, liquid herbal extracts best address all of these factors. This is the reason that American herbalists recommend this form of herbs the most.

Q: What are liquid herbal extracts?
Liquid herbal extracts are herbs that have been processed in such a way that their active constituents (ingredients) are suspended in a liquefied medium, usually alcohol and water. If the alcohol is left in the formulation, an alcohol-

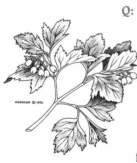

Cramp Bark

containing extract is the result. However, once the constituents have been extracted, the alcohol in the extract can be removed using a heat-free process to produce alcohol-free herbs also. The alcohol-free herbs are then suspended in glycerin to make an alcohol-free extract or suspended in olive oil to create a liquid herbal extract in a softgel.

Q: Why are herbs in liquid herbal extract form preferable over dried herbs in capsule or tablet form?
The success of herbal products as healing agents is dependent upon how active their constituents (ingredients) are when you ingest them. For maximum therapeutic benefits, therefore, it is very important to take herbs in the form that best captures and preserves their active constituents. Liquid herbal extracts achieve this so they are, by far, the most therapeutically beneficial form of herbs available on the market today.

Most herbs in tablet or capsule form are ground months prior to appearing on store shelves. They lose many of their active ingredients both when they are ground and while they are in storage. Herbal tablets also contain fillers, binders and other materials necessary to compress ground herbs into tablet form. Tablets must also be dissolved by the body's digestive system before the herbs can be assimilated. Herbal capsules tend to be better than tablets because they do not contain the extra manufacturing materials and they dissolve easily in the stomach. However, if the body is not digesting and assimilating well, the potential therapeutic benefits of herbs in tablet and capsule form diminishes because the digestive system must break the active constituents free from the fiber and cellulose. Herbs in capsule and tablet form also loose potency as they are exposed to oxygen (capsules oxidize more rapidly than tablets).

Herbs in liquid extract form, on the other hand, contain no fillers, binders, or "extra" ingredients so they are immediately assimilated into the body. Nothing has to be broken down or digested in order for the body to absorb them. In liquid form, the herbs are immediately available for assimilation into the bloodstream, glands and organs. Even a person with poor digestion and assimilation can enjoy maximum benefits from liquid herbal extracts.

Q: You say herbalists recommend liquid herbal extracts over other forms of herbs. Can you explain more?

Herbalists prefer liquid herbal extracts over other forms of herbs for four reasons: freshness, potency, absorption and formulation.

Freshness: As detailed in the previous answer, herbs in liquid herbal extract form retain their freshness and potency much longer than ground herbs in capsule or tablet form. Also, in many instances, using fresh herbs is the only way to deliver the specific properties necessary for healing. Liquid herbal extracts start with fresh herbs that are picked and processed the same day so that the active constituents can be preserved. Capsules, tablets, teas and loose herbs, on the other hand, must first be dried, which saps them of the fresh active constituents necessary for healing. Freshness is also dependent upon how herbs are ground. Super-cold (cryogenic) grinding, done minutes before extraction of the herbs, is effective in preserving all of the herbs' active ingredients because it prevents evaporation of essential oils and degradation of active substances.

Potency: Herbalists have long recognized that potency is not about isolating a single "active constituent". Potency results from the interaction of many constituents within each herb. Herbal products containing a full spectrum of bioavailable constituents promote healing as well as the maintenance of health. Liquid herbal extracts, time and again, deliver more bioavailable constituents than any other herbal supplements.

Absorption: Experience has proven that liquid herbal extracts bypass the digestive process and enter the bloodstream rapidly. This makes them the most effective way for the body to absorb medicinal herbs. Once assimilated, the herbs start working in your body within minutes.

Formulation: Liquid herbal extracts can effectively deliver the healing power of several herbs at once. Clinical experience shows those herbal formulas, comprised of a combination of several herbs, produce better results than single herbs. In a formula, each herb is designed to support a specific body system in a manner that complements the action of other herbs, and the systems they support. Well-designed, time-tested formulations address the body's complete needs.

Q: How are the different forms of liquid herbal extracts made?

Liquid herbal extracts are available in alcohol-containing extracts, alcohol-free extracts and liquid herbal softgels capsules. I advise consumers to pay attention to how different brands of extracts are formulated. Product information of the bottles should give you the information you need.

The most potent and effective extracts, whether they are in alcohol containing, alcohol-free or softgel form, should share three important commonalties. They should all start as alcohol-containing extracts to ensure potency. Second, heat should not be used in their manufacturing processes, as heat is very detrimental to the potency of liquid herbal extracts. Third, all should be produced in such a way to ensure that the herbs contain their full spectrum of active constituents.

Effective alcohol-containing extracts are produced by subjecting herbs, in ground or powdered form, to precise ratios of water and alcohol for specified lengths of time. This is done in order to capture the active constituents of those herbs. Two methods yield the most potent herbal extracts. Fresh, undried herbs are most potent when they are "kinetically macerated". Using this method, herbs are first continuously agitated in an alcohol and water solution for 12 to 24 hours, and then soaked in that same liquid solution for a minimum of two weeks. For dried herbs, the active ingredients are best extracted with the use of a special glass funnel called a "cold-extraction percolator". Using this method, an alcohol and water solution is poured over freshly ground dried herbs in the cold-extraction percolator. Notice in both methods that no heat is used, since heat is very damaging to the potency of the herbs' active ingredients.

Hops

Again, the most effective alcohol-free extracts begin as alcohol-containing extracts per the process explained above. Then, using a heat-free vacuum process, the alcohol is removed. The removal of the alcohol must also be done without the use of heat as heat negatively affects the potency of the extract. Next, glycerin is added to bring the extract back to its original volume. Finally, it is important that a preservative of some sort be added to prevent the growth of microbes. Citric acid, found in citrus fruits, is a safe and natural preservative.

To deliver effective potency, liquid herbal softgels must also begin as alcohol containing extracts as explained above. Then, using a heat-free vacuum process, the alcohol is removed. Olive oil is added to this liquid concentrate to permit its encapsulation into a softgel. A softgel is what encapsulates vitamin E. A dropperful of active constituents of a liquid herbal extract is contained in each softgel.

Q: Is it better to buy liquid herbal extracts or softgels made from fresh herbs or dried herbs?
There is no simple answer to this question. It depends on why you are taking the herbs that you are taking. Nettles, for example, can be used fresh or dried. If you need an herb to increase mineral absorption in your body, dried Nettles offers the most benefits. On the other hand, fresh Nettles offers you optimum hay fever relief because once Nettles is dried, its hay fever-alleviating properties disappear. Certain herbs such as Blue Cohosh, Dong Quai, Goldenseal, and Milk Thistle, are better dried because the drying process modifies and enhances the medicinal action. Other herbs, such as Chamomile, Oat seed, Peppermint and Shepherd's Purse should be processed while fresh in order to preserve their delicate volatile oils and other fragile constituents.

These examples show that whether you choose fresh herbs or dried herbs depends on each herb's specific constituents and the therapeutic goal you are trying to achieve. Therefore, some liquid herbal extracts and softgels are made from fresh herbs and others are made from dried herbs. In some formulas, fresh and dried forms are blended together so that you get the best form of each herb for the specific problems you are addressing. This is where an herbalist's expertise in creating the most effective formulation is effective.

Q: Why are alcohol and water used to make quality liquid herbal extracts?

Alcohol and water are used because both of these substances are necessary to ensure full extraction of all the active ingredients of the herbs. Goldenseal best illustrates this principle. Boiling this root for hours in water will extract its water-soluble properties but will fail to extract hydrastine, its main anti-inflammatory constituent. Only alcohol at a minimum of 60 percent will extract this valuable constituent. The alcohol content in different extracts ranges from as little as 20 percent to as high as 95 percent. The varying amounts of alcohol that are needed for maximum extraction are determined by the properties of the herbs. Vinegar and glycerin cannot replace alcohol as efficient extractive agents.

Q: When the label says an extract has 70 percent alcohol in it, does that mean the remaining 30 percent is herbs and water?

No, it doesn't. One hundred percent of the mixture in the bottle contains herbs. To use an analogy, let's say you stir in one ounce of sugar into four ounces of water. You still have four ounces of water, but it is now sweet. The water is now permeated with sugar, which is no longer visible as a separate ingredient. This analogy holds with herbal formulations. If a particular extract uses 70 percent alcohol and 30 percent water to extract and preserve the herbs, both the 70 percent alcohol and the 30 percent water are imbued with herbs. They hold the herbs just as the water in this example holds the sugar.

Q: I'm alcohol sensitive. How much alcohol will I ingest in an average dose of a liquid herbal extract containing alcohol?

Although some people may be concerned about the amount of alcohol in alcohol-containing liquid herbal extracts, there is little cause for worry. On average, 30 drops of an extract containing 70 percent alcohol (see the label on the bottle for the percentage of alcohol) has the same amount of alcohol as one ripe banana. When we eat fruit, our bodies naturally produce alcohol via the fermentation process in our stomachs. The point I am making here is that most alcohol sensitive people do not quit eating fruit. So if one dosage is only a banana's worth of alcohol, that should not pose a threat to most people.

Q: I still feel that a ripe banana's worth of alcohol is still too much for me. Is there any way I can get the maximum benefits of a liquid herbal extract and avoid the alcohol?

Evaporating the alcohol out of an alcohol-containing liquid herbal extract is best done on a dose-by-dose basis by putting the dose in a hot drink. Do not heat up an entire bottle of herbs, as that would damage the herbs in the extract. Instead, add as many drops of the extract as are recommended per dosage to a cup of boiling water, or, if you wish, to an herbal tea that is naturally caffeine-free. Let the mixture sit for 5-10 minutes. Forty to 60 percent of the alcohol will evaporate during that time. In an extract containing 70 percent alcohol, the remaining alcohol will be about the same as you would find in a third of a ripe banana. Evaporating the alcohol in this manner does not in any way diminish the effectiveness of the herbs in an alcohol-containing extract. Or, you can avoid all alcohol by taking an alcohol-free extract, or an alcohol-free liquid herbal softgel.

Q: Are alcohol-free extracts as potent as alcohol-containing extracts?

As the market stands right now, most alcohol-based extracts are much stronger than alcohol-free extracts. The fact is that most alcohol free extracts only contain a few active constituents and, as such, they are not a good value for the money.

Generally, herbs in liquid herbal extracts made with alcohol are stronger because they have more active constituents available to the user, and they have a longer shelf life as well. One study that I was involved in compared alcohol-free extracts of Goldenseal to alcohol-containing extracts of Goldenseal by measuring the levels of two major active alkaloids in each form of extract. The study verified that there was a direct correlation between the alcohol percentage and the level of alkaloids present. The results showed that the lower the percentage of alcohol equaled lower levels of healing alkaloids in the extracts. In fact, the alcohol-free extracts tested were so low in potency that they were practically useless. According to the study's ratings, you would have needed ten bottles of an alcohol-free extract rated "best" and 256 (yes, that's 256) bottles of an alcohol-free extract rated "worst" to equal one good bottle of alcohol-based extract.

Q: Does this mean there are no potent alcohol-free extracts on the market then?

No, the good news is that one manufacturer, Herbs, Etc., has found a way to produce strong alcohol-free extracts. Two main factors determine if an alcohol-free extract is potent: first, how are the active constituents of the herbs extracted, and second, is heat used in the alcohol-removing process.

When it comes to making alcohol-free extracts, manufacturers are faced with the question of how to effectively extract the active constituents of herbs and make a potent alcohol-free extract at the same time. Most manufacturers, therefore, choose glycerin over alcohol in their extraction processes. The problem is that glycerin does not effectively extract the active constituents, as the study cited in the last question verifies. Capitalizing on these findings, Herbs, Etc. uses alcohol in the extraction of herbs for its alcohol-free extracts. A second problem arises if heat is used in the removal of alcohol to produce alcohol-free herbal extracts as heat kills the active constituents. Herbs, Etc. has found a way around these two issues using alcohol, not glycerin, and then removing the alcohol by a cold, (not hot) extraction process.

A recent study conducted by a renowned Canadian university specializing in Echinacea analysis performed the study confirms the effectiveness of Herbs, Etc.'s manufacturing process. In the study, Echinacea angustifolia in several alcohol-free extracts were analyzed both for water-soluble constituents (caffeic acid derivatives) and alcohol-soluble constituents (isobutylamides). The results showed that the extract made by Herbs, Etc. was three to 20 times stronger than any other leading alcohol-free extracts. A second finding indicated that this new alcohol-free extract had the same amounts per volume of water-soluble and alcohol-soluble constituents as the best alcohol-containing extract.

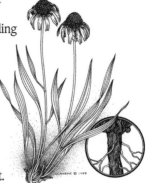

Echinacea angustifolia

Q: I have read about herbs that are "standardized". What is standardization?

Standardization of herbal products occurs when a specific amount of one "active constituent" in an herb is artificially manipulated to be at a certain level. In the last few years there has been an ongoing trend in the herbal industry to "standardize" herbal products. This phenomenon is occurring principally because of two strong influences. First, medical doctors are being drawn to herbs by patients who are growing uncomfortable with synthetic drugs. Patients are requesting products with fewer side effects but with equally effective natural properties. Coming from an orthodox, pharmaceutically-driven framework, doctors feel more comfortable when they can recommend products that have "active constituents" in measurable and consistent amounts. Thus, they are encouraging the standardization of herbs. Second, in response to pressure from medical doctors to bring herbs in line with how drugs are standardized, some herb companies are also behind developing such products.

Q: Is the standardization of herbs valid in your opinion? Does it increase the healing potential of herbs?

In my opinion, standardization runs counter to the holistic view that each herb is an ecosystem that combines all of its parts to heal and balance our bodies. I strongly believe that, in most instances, using whole herbs is superior to standardizing fragments of herbs.

In support of this point of view, I point to the issues that are outstanding in the debate over this topic. The biggest problem with standardizing herbal products becomes apparent when one looks at all the constituents found in any given herb. Just which of an herb's numerous constituents should be chosen as being the effective one? The truth is we do not know what the active constituents are in 98 percent of the herbs that are available on the market.

Research on Echinacea illustrates why the question of "Which one of the many constituents is the active constituent?" is still unanswered. In the late 1970s and the early 1980s, researchers concluded that the polysaccharides in Echinacea had many immunostimulating activities. Based on this research, European companies standardized their Echinacea products to achieve a specific amount of polysaccharides (usually labeled as echinacosides). Subsequent research revealed that alcohol soluble constituents were even more effective in supporting the immune system than the polysaccharides. It doesn't stop there. Year by year, even more new Echinacea compounds have been isolated and identified.

An overview of the process of trying to standardize Valerian also provides another case in point. First, it was thought that the essential oils were the active constituents of Valerian. But when the essential oils alone were administered to people, they achieved only partial results. Then it was thought that valepotriates were the active ingredients until testing revealed only partial results again. Still later, valerenic acid was thought to be the active ingredient. More testing, same results. The irony is that each testing process actually supports the fact that the whole herb gives better results than any fraction of the herb.

The second issue that comes up as to whether standardized herbs are the way to go is that the standardization of a few effective products has been assumed to be possible for all herbs. Yes, there have been a handful of standardized herbal products that have been shown to be effective in certain situations. For instance, Milk Thistle with standardized silymarin levels is effective for serious liver diseases. However, if one is using Milk Thistle as a liver protectant, a whole seed liquid extract protects the liver just as well as a standardized extract—at a fraction of the cost of a standardized extract. In addition, the whole seed contains many other innate substances not present in the standardized product that help support the healing of the liver.

The successful standardization of about a half dozen herbs (Bilberry, Ephedra, Ginkgo, Grape Seed extract, Gugulipid and Milk Thistle) is simply not applicable to all herbs, or applicable for all their uses. Remember that in over 98 percent of herbs, we simply do not know what the active constituents are. Key questions that emerge out of all these research projects include: "To which active constituent should an herb be standardized?" and "Does standardizing certain constituents in herbs make them better products?" The answers are still inconclusive.

Q: How long do herbs in different forms retain their effectiveness?

Form	Shelf Life
Powdered Herbs	1-6 months
Tea Bags	1-6 months
Herbal Capsules	1-12 months
Whole dried Leaves	2-12 months
Herbal Tablets	2-24 months
Whole dried Root	1-3 years
Liquid Herbal Extract Softgels	3 years
Alcohol-free Liquid Extracts	3 years
Alcohol-containing Liquid Extracts	at least 7 years

This chart points out that the more an herb is ground or reduced in size, the more rapidly it will lose its beneficial properties. In general, whole herbs tend to retain their medicinal properties or "shelf life" longer than other forms of herbs. This chart also shows that liquid herbal extracts maintain a longer shelf life than other forms of herbs. Once the herbs are extracted in a liquid medium, very little evaporation, oxidation or degradation of active constituents occurs.

Q: How should I care for liquid herbal extracts or softgels to keep them fresh?

For optimum shelf life of alcohol-free or alcohol-containing extracts, including softgels, I suggest a three point approach. First, keep your liquid herbal extracts away from sunlight/windows. Second, keep your extracts away from hot temperatures, such as storing them in the glove compartment of your car in the summertime. Especially softgels, as they will melt. Third, keep bottle caps firmly closed. Unopened bottles of alcohol-free liquid herbal extracts have a three-year shelf life. Once opened, it is recommended that alcohol-free extracts be used or discarded within six months. This precaution is necessary to prevent bacterial contamination. This six-month shelf life for an unopened bottle of alcohol-free extract can be extended by another six months if you refrigerate the extract.

Alcohol-containing extracts, opened or unopened, have a shelf life of at least seven years if the recommendations made above are followed. Refrigeration is not necessary. Softgels will last three years, opened or unopened. No refrigeration is necessary.

Q: How can I tell if an extract has gone "bad"?

In my experience with alcohol-containing liquid herbal extracts, it is rare for extracts not to last for years when they are stored properly. The only exception to this rule that I have found is with extracts containing Ephedra (Ma Huang). If you have an extract containing Ephedra and you see that the herbs are clumping together in the bottle or the dropper, I recommend discarding the bottle.

With alcohol-free liquid herbal extracts, the product should contain citric acid, a natural preservative. Should the product not contain a preservative such as citric acid, smell the product. If the product has a musty odor or seems to have any growth, immediately discard the product. Even with a citric acid containing alcohol-free product, discard the product within six months of opening it or after one year if the product has been refrigerated.

Q: Does it matter if the herbs I take are organic?

As an herbalist concerned about our environment, I strongly recommend that herbal consumers choose certified organically grown herbs.

First, choosing organically cultivated herbs helps lessen over-harvesting of herbs in the wild. For example, Echinacea and Goldenseal, among other herbs, are facing extinction unless we start cultivating these plants. Second, certified organic farmers make sure they have crops year after year by not compromising their land for short-term gain. Therefore, by buying organic, you support renewing the land. Third, certified organic farmers are inspected by a third-party certifying agency, insuring that the farmers utilize sustainable, chemical-free and pesticide-free farming techniques. This means that organic herbs truly support your healing as well as help preserve the health of our planet.

Q: What should I look for when I buy liquid herbal extracts or softgels?

1.)Look for sufficient alcohol amount and cold processing. Be aware of the production process that the herbs have gone through. Choose alcohol-containing extracts with a minimum of 20 percent alcohol. The alcohol acts as a preservative and prevents contamination of the herbs by fungus, bacteria and viruses. Alcohol levels higher than 20 percent are needed to extract many different herbs. For example, Milk Thistle and Cayenne need at least 95 percent alcohol in order to extract the active constituents. Echinacea and Goldenseal require 70 percent while herbs like Peppermint and Chamomile require a much lower alcohol percentage. When extracts are made from whole herbs ground cryogenically (cold grinding) minutes prior to extraction, no constituents are destroyed by friction-induced heat during the grinding process. Cold process kinetic maceration for fresh herbs or cold process percolation for dried herbs yields more active ingredients in finished extracts than in herbs processed by using other methods.

In alcohol-free extracts or softgels, make sure that the extract was originally extracted with alcohol, then the alcohol was removed without the use of heat. Citric acid should be added as a natural preservative. When choosing softgels, ensure that the extraction was done using alcohol and that the alcohol was then removed.

2.)Buy organically grown herbs. Choose herbal extracts made from certified organically grown herbs when possible. When certified organically grown herbs are not available, choose wild harvested herbs picked in regions that are not exposed to pesticides, herbicides, or chemical fertilizers.

3.)Choose liquid herbal extracts in formulas. Choose herbal formula combinations, especially when you are not quite sure which single herb(s) to choose. The formulas listed in this book are available in alcohol-containing extracts, alcohol-free extracts and liquid herbal softgels, and have been blended, tested and approved by Medical Herbalist, Daniel Gagnon.

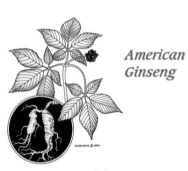

American Ginseng

Chapter 4:
Taking Medicinal Herbal Extracts

Q: Is it better to choose herbal formulas instead of single herbs?

To get the results you hope to achieve, it is important to choose the herbs that best address your specific health concerns. This book lists both single herbal extracts and formulas, as both are effective healing agents.

I generally favor formulas because I feel they offer greater health benefits, greater affordability and greater convenience. For example, if you look in the **Health Condition Index** of this book under arthritis, you will see that several single extracts (including Devil's Claw and Meadowsweet) and two formulas (Arthrotonic™ and Herbaprofen™) are recommended. If you then read the description of each of the single extracts in the **Herbal Directory** (Chapter 7), you will see that each herb works in a specific way to alleviate arthritis. For example, Devil's Claw works on arthritic inflammation and helps the liver excrete waste products that may contribute to inflammation. Meadowsweet works over the long term to relieve pain and also supports the kidneys to excrete waste products that aggravate inflammation. As you can see, deep knowledge of botanical medicine, the body's physiology and your particular symptoms are required to distinguish which herb is the most appropriate herb to take.

On the other hand, when you read the description of the formula Arthrotonic™, you will see that it combines Devil's Claw and nine other herbs, which all perform specific functions to relieve the symptoms of arthritis and help the body get healthy again. The formula Herbaprofen™ combines Jamaican Dogwood, Meadowsweet and seven other herbs, again all with specific functions for, in this case, relieving pain. The guesswork of determining which single extracts to take has been eliminated. The cost of buying one or two formulas versus buying all of the single extracts included in each formula is significantly less. The level of support for your arthritis is greatly amplified because a formula is stronger than the sum of its herbal parts. Each herb complements the others and together they form a strong coalition to support the body in its quest for health.

Q: Do I use herbs differently when I have an acute condition, as opposed to when I have a chronic condition?

During an **acute phase** of a health condition (rapid onset, severe symptoms, short course, as in colds or flu), it is desirable to take herbs on a frequent basis to maintain a high level of the herbs' active constituents in the bloodstream. This way, the herbs' constituents constantly bathe the affected tissues. If the therapeutic level falls off, the invading microorganisms or the inflammation threatening the tissues will flare. Your body then has to redouble its efforts to get the affected tissues back to normal. Taking care of the acute phase quickly and completely prevents the problem from becoming chronic or recurrent.

During a **chronic phase** of a disease (long duration, ongoing or recurring symptoms, as in arthritis), it is important to take herbs on a regular basis over a longer period of time in order to offer the challenged tissues healing support. For chronic phases, you need to supply the affected tissues with nutrients and herbal substances on a daily basis so that the tissues can heal and resume their normal functions.

Valeria

Arthritis again provides us with a clear example of how herbs address acute versus chronic phases of a health condition. In the chronic phase of arthritis, a person will have stiffness and dull pain in the joints; whereas during an acute flare-up, inflammation, sharper pain, as well as swelling, will be present. Both phases should be addressed, but in different ways. In an acute flare-up, the strategy is to decrease inflammation and get rid of the waste products that are contributing to the inflammation. This requires frequent dosages. During a chronic phase, the strategy is to stabilize and help repair the tissues, and prevent future flare-ups. This requires larger dosages, taken fewer times a day, over longer periods of time.

Q: What is the best time of day to take liquid herbal extracts?

In most instances, I suggest taking extracts between meals, apart from eating food. This way, extracts don't have to compete with food and the digestive process and the constituents rapidly enter the bloodstream and immediately start the healing process. A few herbs, however, are better taken before meals. For example, bitter herbs help tone up the stomach and increase production of hydrochloric acid and other digestive enzymes. Others, like sleep aid herbs, are better taken one hour before bedtime to permit relaxation and more restful sleep. Pay attention to the dosage notation under each herb in the **Herbal Directory** (Chapter 7) for specific directions on timing.

Q: How do I know when to stop taking an extract?

Herbs work in an individual way within each body. Some herbs act very quickly, while others take more time to balance, nourish and support body systems. Certain herbs are best taken for a short time (one to three weeks) while other herbs will yield their best results when they are taken for longer periods (one to six months or longer). When duration is specifically important, it will be noted in the dosage recommendations in the **Herbal Directory** (Chapter 7).

The following considerations determine duration. In general, the stronger the herb, the shorter the length of time it should be taken. Examples of these strong herbs include Chaparral, Goldenseal, Lomatium and Uva Ursi. Other herbs, such as Ginkgo, Hawthorn, Oat Seed and St. John's Wort, must be taken for a least one month before they even begin to share their healing qualities with us.

Formulas designed to be taken during acute health conditions, such as Goldenseal/Echinacea Complex for colds and flu, should be taken for shorter amounts of time. On the other hand, formulas aimed at chronic problems, such as Deprezac™ for depression, and Deep Health™ for deep immune system support, require longer periods of ingestion. Their benefits accrue over time.

When you are treating a problem that has existed for a long time, it is sometimes helpful to alternate between two formulas. Using acne as an example, take Acnetonic™ for one month and then take Dermatonic™ for one month. Start again with the Acnetonic™ and keep cycling every other month until the problem is resolved. If duration is not indicated, then take the herb until symptoms cease. If you are in doubt, consult a knowledgeable herbalist, a naturopath or primary care physician. Keep in mind that herbs are medicine and recommended dosages should not be exceeded.

Q: Since I am dealing with several different health conditions, what is the best way to take herbs for more than one problem at once?
When taking different herbs for different health problems, there are four points to keep in mind. These guidelines are applicable to all age groups.

1) Go to the root of your problems rather than just treating separate symptoms. For example, a person may experience difficulty sleeping, sour stomach, cystitis, sinusitis and nervousness. If you treat each symptom as a separate problem, you will need herbs for the urinary, digestive and respiratory systems, as well as herbs for the nervous system. What may be needed instead are herbs targeted at stress. Or it may be that the best system to strengthen is the digestive system if that is where the root of the different symptoms is centered. When the root cause is addressed with appropriate herbs, then the other remaining symptoms will disappear.

2) Take herbs for different problems at different times. Take herbs for the same problem at the same time. For example, if you want to take Arthrotonic™ for arthritis and Feverfew for migraine headaches, I suggest that you take them at least fifteen minutes apart. On the other hand, if you are taking different herbs for the same problem, such as Dandelion, Burdock and Nettle for skin problems, they can be combined and taken at the same time.

Milk Thistle

See item 4 below regarding guidelines for how many extracts to take at once.

3) Take herbs at least fifteen minutes apart.
See item 2 above.

4) It is usually best to address no more than three health problems at once. Let's say you are taking herbs for asthma, arthritis and migraines, but you also suffer from skin rashes and chronic fatigue. First, decide which three health conditions to address, and then take the herbs for those conditions at least fifteen minutes apart. It is okay to take a single extract, like Feverfew, for your migraines, and also to take combinations, like Adrenotonic™ for your asthma, and Arthrotonic™ for your arthritis. For best results, also take these combinations apart from each other.

Q: Can I take herbal extracts at the same time I am taking conventional drugs?
In many instances taking herbs at the same time as conventional drugs will actually support and heal the body faster and more thoroughly. For example, taking immune stimulating herbs while a person is on antibiotics is recommended, because these herbs will strengthen the immune system and prevent relapses after the round of antibiotics is done. In other instances it is best not to take herbal extracts at the same time as conventional drugs. For example, I do not recommend taking antidepressant drugs and herbal antidepressants at the same time. Be aware that when herbs are combined with drugs, they can increase the action of the drugs. Consult a knowledgeable herbalist, a naturopath or primary care physician when combining any medications.

Q: Why do some extracts taste so awful?
Don't let taste keep you from enjoying the healing benefits of herbs. In our society, we are addicted to two basic tastes: salty and sweet. But there are three other tastes that are equally important in maintaining health: sour, bitter and pungent. These tastes, when taken as herbs or foods, initiate body reactions that help restore health. For example bitter herbs, such as Barberry, help tone the stomach. Pungent tasting herbs, such as Turmeric, help tone the liver. It is important to remember that herbs, even though they may not taste salty or sweet, put us in touch with nature's pure energy to assist us in our quest for health. When the taste of herbs is a major

inconvenience, the benefits and effectiveness of liquid herbal extracts are available in the convenience of softgels.

Q: What is the best way to disguise the taste of liquid herbal extracts?

The easiest way to disguise the taste of liquid herbal extracts is to take them in softgel form because they bypass the taste buds. The best way to take alcohol-containing or alcohol-free liquid herbal extracts without affecting their healing properties is to put them in eight ounces of water, juice, and/or herbal tea, as long as the tea doesn't contain caffeine. Although some people prefer to put undiluted liquid herbal extracts directly in their mouths, putting extracts in some form of liquid is easier for most people. Herbs taken for digestion are best taken in only two or three ounces of water so that you can taste the bitterness of the herbs. It is the bitterness that enhances digestion.

Q: Can I give liquid herbal extracts to my children?

There are four things you must be aware of with children and liquid herbal extracts.

1) *Children should be at least one year old before they are given herbs.* Children under a year old should only be given extracts under the supervision of a knowledgeable herbalist or primary care physician (medical doctor, naturopath, acupuncturist, etc.). In a few instances in the **Herbal Directory** (Chapter 7), reference is made to certain herbs which can be given to babies. These are Chamomile, Fennel, Pau D'Arco and Stomach Tonic™. See specific dosage instructions under these listings.

2) *A child's dosage is a fraction of the adult dosage.* If an extract calls for a 20-drop dose for an adult, adjust the dosage by giving two drops per year of age to a child. For example, a three-year-old child would take six drops of the extract (20 = 2 drops x 3 years old = 6 drops). If the extract calls for a 10-drop dose for an adult, adjust the dosage by giving one drop per year of age. Therefore, a three-year-old child would take three drops of the extract (10 = 1 drop x 3 years old = 3 drops). California Poppy, Horsetail, Passionflower and Red Clover, as noted in the **Herbal Directory** (Chapter 7), are exceptions to this rule. See specific dosage instructions under these listings.

A second way to figure out a child's dosage is to divide the adult dosage by 150 pounds and multiply the answer by the weight of the child. For example, take an adult dosage of 30 drops and divide by 150 pounds = 2/10 of a drop, multiplied by the weight of a 30 pound child = 6 drops.

3) *If the child is of slight build or is underweight for his/her age,* determine the correct dosage by the weight of the child according to the formula above.

4) *If the child has a weak constitution, i.e. is frail, recuperating from an illness or is in any weakened state,* cut the usual child's dosage by 25-50 percent. Gauge dosage according to effectiveness.

Q: How can I get my child to take liquid herbal extracts?
Alcohol-free liquid herbal extracts have a pleasant citrus flavor. Putting the drops in orange juice is the easiest way to give an herbal extract to a child, because it disguises the taste. Other juices may also do the trick.

Q: Can I give liquid herbal extracts to my pets? How much should I give them?
I have found over the years that pets respond very favorably to extracts. However, in the same way that you need to adjust dosages for children, care should be taken to adjust dosages for animals. The general rule is to give two drops per 10 pounds of weight. The best way to give extracts to pets is to mix it in their food. It is not necessary to evaporate the alcohol, as the amount of alcohol in a dose is too small to hurt them.

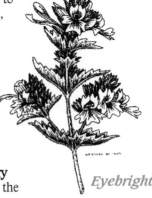

Eyebright

Q: How many drops should I take?
For best results follow the dosages suggested in the **Herbal Directory** (Chapter 7) under the appropriate herb.

Q: How many drops are in a one-ounce bottle of alcohol-containing or alcohol-free extracts? How many drops are in a softgel?

There are approximately 1,200 drops in a one-ounce bottle of an alcohol-containing or alcohol-free liquid herbal extract. Each softgel contains the equivalent of 30 drops of a liquid herbal extract.

Q: How do I compare regular herbal capsules to liquid herbal extracts or softgels? How do milligrams compare to drops?

It is difficult to compare regular herbal capsules to liquid herbal extracts, especially when it comes to issues concerning assimilation and potency. With regular herbal capsules, the body first has to break down plant fibers, and then digest and assimilate the plant constituents. If a person taking capsules has any digestive problems, breaking down and assimilating the herbs will be incomplete. In the case of liquid extracts or softgels, the body assimilates them more rapidly and thoroughly.

On the issue of potency, regular herbal capsules lose potency through evaporation, oxidation and degradation, both in the manufacturing process and every day that they sit on the shelf. On the other hand, because liquid herbal extracts are processed immediately after harvesting and their active constituents are preserved, liquid herbal extracts or softgels will keep their potency for a minimum of three years. Capsules cannot rival that. Each softgel contains liquid herbal extract concentrate and offers the benefits of taking approximately one and one-half capsules of ground herbs. Therefore, the following equivalencies are at best approximate.

25 mg = 1 drop

50 mg = 2 drops

500 mg = 20 drops

One softgel = 30 drops

One dropperful = 30 drops

Approximately forty dropperfuls per bottle=1200 drops

(a one-ounce bottle)

Chapter 5:
Deciding When to Avoid Certain Herbs

Q: If I am pregnant or breast-feeding, what precautions should I use when taking herbs?

Here is a list of herbs and herbal formulas that should be avoided during pregnancy and breast-feeding unless specifically recommended by a knowledgeable herbalist, naturopath or other primary care physician. Because some herbs have a direct influence on the uterus the most common contraindication is when pregnancy is involved. Other herbs are contraindicated while breast-feeding because some of the herbs' constituents may migrate into and through the milk to the infant. I have also included laxatives in this list even though they are not found in this book. Laxatives may have undesirable side effects for pregnant or breast-feeding women. Be sure to note the recommendations and contraindications listed with each herb in the **Herbal Directory** (Chapter 7).

Herbs to Avoid in Pregnancy
Single extracts and formulas are listed separately

Single herbs not to be taken during pregnancy
Ashwagandha
Barberry
Black Cohosh (Not in the first seven months.)
Blue Cohosh (Not in the first seven months.)
California Poppy
Catnip
Chaparral
Dong Quai
Ephedra (Ma Huang)
Feverfew
Goldenseal
Hyssop
Juniper
Kava
Licorice
Lobelia
Lomatium
Motherwort

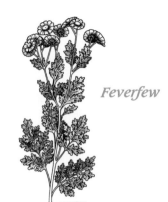

Feverfew

WERNEKE © 1993

37

Myrrh
Osha
Pennyroyal
Pleurisy Root
Red Clover
Shepherd's Purse
Turmeric
Uva Ursi
Vitex
Yarrow

Laxatives to be avoided: Aloin (an aloe extract), Buckthorn, Cascara Sagrada, Rhubarb root and Senna although not found in this book should be avoided in pregnancy.

Formulas not to be taken during pregnancy

Acnetonic™
Adrenotonic™
Arthrotonic™
Bionic Tonic™
Cardiotonic™
Cholesterotonic™
Congest Free™
Cran-Bladder ReLeaf™
Cycle 1 Estrotonic™
Cycle 2 Progestonic™
Decongestonic™
Dermatonic™
Digestonic™
Essiac Tonic
Goldenseal/Echinacea Complex
HB Pressure Tonic™
Herbaprofen™
Kava Cool Complex™
Kidalin®
Kidney Tonic™
Liver Tonic™
Lymphatonic™
Menopautonic™
Montezuma's ReLeaf™
Monthly ReLeaf™
M-Roid ReLeaf™
Nervine Tonic™
Osha Root Complex Syrup (Not in the first three months)
Para-Free™
Phytocillin™
PMS ReLeaf™

WERNEKE © 1993

Goldenseal

Respiratonic™
Smoke Free Drops™
Stomach Tonic™
Vein Tonic™
Yeast ReLeaf™

Herbs to Avoid While Breast-Feeding:
Single extracts and formulas are listed together

Black Cohosh
Congest Free™
Decongestonic™
Ephedra (Ma Huang)
Herbaprofen™
Kava
Kava Cool Complex™
Licorice
Para-Free™

Laxatives to be avoided: Aloin (an aloe extract), Buckthorn, Cascara Sagrada, Rhubarb root and Senna although not found in this book, should be avoided while breast-feeding.

Q: What are "contraindications"?
Considering the hundreds of medicinal herbs available, not many have contraindications. The word "contraindication" is defined by *Tabor's Cyclopedic Medical Dictionary* (1977) as, "any symptom or circumstance indicating the inappropriateness of a form of treatment otherwise advisable." Some herbs are contraindicated during acute inflammation because they can actually cause more inflammation at that stage of an illness. For example, Juniper is contraindicated during acute urinary tract infection, as it can increase the inflammation that is already present. Other herbs are contraindicated with prescribed medications or in preexisting conditions. When a contraindication is noted in the **Herbal Directory** (Chapter 7), it means you must either alter your dosage as recommended, or not take that herb if you have the condition that is contraindicated. Pay strict attention to the directions given with each herb.

Q: What is a "side effect"? Do herbs have side effects like drugs?
Few herbs have negative drug-like side effects. This is one of the primary reasons that so many people are turning to herbs as their preferred mode of treatment.

Tabor's Cyclopedic Medical Dictionary defines a side effect as, "the action or effect, usually of a drug, other than that desired." In some instances side effects of herbs aren't damaging but they simply have an effect that you should be aware of. For example, some herbs may change the color or smell of the urine.

However, there are a few herbs listed in this book that may cause undesirable side effects, especially if they are taken in larger amounts than recommended. In addition, there is always the possibility that a few individuals may have unpredictable reactions to herbs.

Q: What are "warnings"?

An informed consumer can exercise educated choices. This section is aimed at providing additional information to favor the safe use of herbs. *Webster's Encyclopedic Unabridged Dictionary* defines warning as "serving to give notice, advice or intimation to a person of danger, possible harm or anything else unfavorable". A few of the herbs listed in this book may cause undesirable outcomes or may interact with drugs in a negative way.

Pay close attention to the dosage directions and all applicable notations regarding contra-indications, side effects and warning given with each herb in the **Herbal Directory** (Chapter 7). The following lists summarize contraindications, possible side effects and warnings of herbs:

General Contraindications of Herbs:

Arnica — do not use on open wounds or broken skin

Ashwagandha — do not use with barbiturates

California Poppy — do not use with MAO-inhibitors

Cayenne — do not use on broken skin or near eyes

Chaparral — do not use with pre-existing kidney disease or liver conditions (hepatitis, cirrhosis)

Congest Free™ — do not use with anorexia, bulimia or glaucoma

Dandelion root — do not use with blockage of the bile ducts, acute gallbladder inflammation, and intestinal blockage

Decongestonic™ — do not use with anorexia, bulimia or glaucoma

Devil's Claw — do not use with gastric and duodenal ulcers

Dong Quai — do not use during acute inflammation

of uterine, vaginal, ovarian or prostatic tissues

Ephedra (Ma Huang) — do not use with anorexia, bulimia or glaucoma

Fo-ti — do not use when diarrhea is present

Gentian — do not use with gastric and duodenal ulcers, gastric irritation and inflammation

Ginseng, Chinese Kirin Red — do not use with thyroid disease, high blood pressure, hyperglycemia, or in insomnia

Hawthorn — do not use with digitalis

Hops — do not use with depression

Horsetail — do not use with cardiac or renal dysfunction

Juniper — do not use with acute urinary tract inflammation, stomach inflammation or serious kidney disease

Kava — do not use with alcohol or barbiturates

Kava Cool Complex™ — do not use with alcohol or barbiturates

Licorice — do not use with high blood pressure from sodium retention or hypokalemia (low blood potassium level)

Mullein/Garlic Ear Drops — do not use with perforated eardrums

Myrrh — do not use with overt kidney disease or excessive uterine bleeding

St. John's Wort — do not use with antidepressants

Turmeric — do not use with bile duct obstruction, stomach/duodenal ulcers or hyperacidity

Uva Ursi — do not use with a history of kidney disorders, irritated digestive conditions and with acidic urine or in conjunction with remedies which produce acidic urine

Vitex — do not use with oral contraceptives

Possible Side Effects of Herbs:

Arnica — may cause skin rash (allergic dermatitis) in sensitive persons, or with prolonged use

Bionic Tonic™ — may cause insomnia

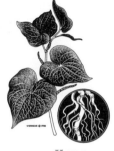

Kava

Black Cohosh — excessive use may cause occasional gastrointestinal discomfort, mild frontal headache, dizziness, impaired vision, vertigo, nausea, vomiting, and/or impaired circulation

Blue Cohosh — may cause mid-cycle spotting & cramping in sensitive women

Cayenne — may cause stomach or intestinal irritation

Chlorophyll Concentrate™ — dark green stools may occur

Congest Free™ — may cause insomnia, nervousness, loss of appetite, nausea, tremor, or high blood pressure

Cran-Bladder ReLeaf™ — peculiar urine smell and color may occur

Decongestonic™ — may cause insomnia, nervousness, loss of appetite, nausea, tremor, or high blood pressure

Ephedra (Ma Huang) — may cause insomnia, nervousness, loss of appetite, nausea, tremor, or high blood pressure

Feverfew — mouth ulceration or gastric disturbance may occur

Ginseng, Chinese Kirin Red — may cause insomnia

HB Pressure Tonic™ — may cause low blood pressure

Hops — may cause depression (with long term usage)

Juniper — may aggravate stomach or kidney inflammation

Kava — large amounts over an extended period of time may cause skin rash

Kava Cool Complex™ — large amounts over an extended period of time may cause skin rash

Kidney Tonic™ — peculiar urine smell and color may occur

Licorice — large amounts over an extended period of time may cause high blood pressure, water retention, headache and vertigo

Lobelia — may cause nausea and vomiting

Lomatium — may cause skin rash

Myrrh — large amounts may cause diarrhea and irritation of the kidneys

Pleurisy Root — may cause nausea and vomiting

Shepherd's Purse — large doses of extract may cause heart palpitations

St. John's Wort — may cause increased photo-sensitivity(which may lead to skin rash) in fair-skinned individuals

Uva Ursi — may cause stomach irritation

Wild Yam — large doses of the extract may cause vomiting

Warnings for Herbs:

Arnica — FOR EXTERNAL USE ONLY. If the skin becomes irritated, cease use

Ashwagandha — may potentiate the effects of barbiturates

Black Walnut — not for prolonged use

Blueberry — not useful in insulin-dependent diabetes

California Poppy — may potentiate the effects of MAO-inhibitors

Cardiotonic™ — not useful for damaged heart where the damage is termed organic. Works best for functional heart problems (i.e., angina)

Cayenne — if the skin becomes irritated, cease use

Chaparral — discontinue use if nausea, fever, fatigue or jaundice (e.g. dark or yellow discoloration of the eyes) should occur

Congest Free™ — seek advice from a health care practitioner prior to use if you have high blood pressure, heart or thyroid disease, diabetes, difficulty in urination due to prostate enlargement or if taking an MAO-inhibitor. Reduce or discontinue use if nervousness, tremor, sleeplessness, loss of appetite, nausea or high blood pressure occur. Do not take for more than six weeks in succession

Decongestonic™ — seek advice from a health care practitioner prior to use if you have high blood pressure, heart or thyroid disease, diabetes, difficulty in urination due to prostate enlargement or if taking an MAO-inhibitor. Reduce or discontinue use if nervousness, tremor, sleeplessness, loss of appetite, nausea or high blood pressure occur. Do not take for more than six weeks in succession

Deprezac™ — not effective for bi-polar syndrome and/or for any other severe pathological depressive states.

Ephedra — seek advice from a health care practitioner prior to use if you have high blood pressure, heart or thyroid disease, diabetes, difficulty in urination due to prostate enlargement or if taking an MAO-inhibitor. Reduce or discontinue use if nervousness, tremor, sleeplessness, loss of appetite, nausea or high blood pressure occurs. Do not take for more than six weeks in succession

Goldenseal — use until the inflammatory stage goes away, then discontinue use. Not for long term use. Do not exceed recommended dose

....

Hawthorn — may potentiate the effects of digitalis, consult primary care practitioner prior to use with digitalis. Not useful for damaged heart where the damage is termed organic. Works best for functional heart problems (i.e., angina)

HB Pressure Tonic™ — monitor your blood pressure to make sure the herbal treatment is effective for you

Ivy Itch ReLeaf™ — FOR EXTERNAL USE ONLY

Juniper — do not use for more than six weeks in succession. Do not exceed recommend dose

Kava — may potentiate the effects of alcohol or barbituates. Chronic situations may require long term use. Do not exceed recommended dose. If skin rash occurs, cease use

Kava Cool Complex™ — may potentiate the effects of alcohol or barbituates. Chronic situations may require long term use. Do not exceed recommended dose. If skin rash occurs, cease use

Licorice — may potentiate potassium depletion of thiazide diuretics, stimulant laxatives, cardiac glycosides or cortisol. Prolonged use is not recommended

Lobelia — excessive amount slows heart beat and depresses respiration

Lomatium — if skin rash occurs, cease use

Marshmallow — may cause delayed absorption of other drugs taken at the same time

Mullein/Garlic Ear Drops — FOR EXTERNAL USE ONLY. Do not use in ears with perforated eardrums.

Pau D'Arco — for babies less than six months old, use EXTERNALLY only

Phytocillin™ — if infection persists longer than three days or a fever is present, seek the advice of a primary care practitioner

Propolis — should not be used internally by those with known reactions to bees or bee products, such as bee pollen or honey

Shepherd's Purse — if prolonged significant or unusual bleeding occurs, seek medical attention. Individuals with a history of kidney stones should use cautiously

St. John's Wort — may potentiate the effects of antidepressants. Although photosensitivity in human beings is rare, fair-skinned individuals should avoid excessive exposure to UV irriadiation (e.g. sunlight, tanning) Do not use while taking any prescription drugs without the advice of your primary care practitioner

Uva Ursi — not for prolonged use without consulting a primary care practitioner

Vitex — may counteract the effectiveness of birth control pills

Wild Cherry — not for long term use. Do not exceed recommended dose

Yellow Dock — use cautiously when a history of kidney stones is present

Q: Are there precautions around taking herbs for people who are taking prescription, over-the-counter medication or belong to a specific age group?

Yes, there are two points to keep in mind. Is the person taking herbs also being treated with prescription or over-the-counter medications? Or is the person elderly or very young?

1) *If you are taking conventional medication for a health problem, be aware that taking herbs that work on the same medical condition may increase the effect of the drugs.* For example, if you are taking medication to lower your blood pressure and you start taking herbs that do the same thing, you may find that your blood pressure decreases too much. Always monitor the results of taking any medications with your doctor and/or a person knowledgeable about herbs.

2) *For children, especially those under the age of five, and also for adults over the age of 70, special care should be taken when administering herbs.* Children and the elderly may be susceptible either to diarrhea or to excessive stimulation from certain herbs. Therefore it is important to start with smaller dosages and to monitor the reaction. You will find that in most instances everything will be normal. But in a few cases, diarrhea, skin rash, or other symptoms may occur, indicating the need to lessen dosages or to stop giving herbs altogether.

Q. Should I tell my doctor I am taking herbs?

I think it is important to let him/her know what you are taking. While some doctors believe that herbs are dangerous or, conversely, have no effects, other doctors may already be knowledgeable. Many medical doctors are aware of the use of herbs as medicine, but they are unsure where to find accurate, objective and useful information. Sharing this book with your doctor may be helpful to both of you. Education is the key, and this book is an excellent source of information.

Chapter 6:

Targeting Herbs for Specific Complaints

Q: What does "targeting" herbs mean?

"Targeting" means using the most therapeutically focused herb at a specific time for a precise health problem. The herbal recommendations in this chapter were born out of my frustration that most sources of information on herbs do not differentiate clearly between various herbs suggested for a particular health problem. With the image of darts hitting a target in mind, I see each herb as a dart which gives you higher numbers of points the closer you get to using its main strengths at the right time in the course of a disease. Hitting the "bullseye" is when you derive the maximum benefit from an herb.

In relation to treating colds and flu, Goldenseal provides us with an example of how targeting is a tool that gives you stronger, faster and longer lasting results. Presently, most Goldenseal consumed in America in herbal products are used either for the prevention of colds and flu, or for the very beginning phases of colds and flu. Taking Goldenseal for these purposes is simply hitting the outer ring of the target, because only 10 percent to 40 percent of Goldenseal's therapeutic benefits are being tapped. The rest of Goldenseal's benefits are being wasted. Goldenseal hits the bullseye when you use it to combat inflammation that often starts on day three of a cold. The most benefits are derived when Goldenseal is used with inflammation of mucous membranes that has been present for a few days or more.

How to get the most out of this chapter:

Refer to the **Herbal Directory** (Chapter 7) for a description of the healing actions, dosage recommendations, contraindications, possible side effects and warnings, when applicable, for each herb. *Pay special attention to the fact that several of the herbs recommended in these charts are contraindicated in pregnancy and some are contraindicated in breast feeding.*

Herbs for Skin Problems

Skin problems can occur due to a multitude of factors including diet, stress, allergies, contact with irritating substances and even monthly hormonal changes. Many of the drugs used for skin problems suppress symptoms so that the existing problem tends to recur after the drugs are discontinued. In order to rectify skin problems, you need to change how your body processes and eliminates waste products. In holistic herbal therapy, it is said that there is a ten to one ratio between the time an existing problem has been present and the time that it takes to heal the condition. For example, if you have had psoriasis for twenty years, it may take up to two years for your skin to be problem-free. So, be aware that it may take a few weeks to many months to change your pattern but it is possible with persistence.

Symptoms	Recommended Herbs	
	Singles	*Formulas*
Dry flaky skin, eczema, psoriasis	Pleurisy Root	Dermatonic™
Oozy, wet skin, eczema, psoriasis	Dandelion	Dermatonic™
Acne, especially for teens eating fatty foods and sugar	Burdock	Acnetonic™
Acne and herpes around lips, worse around menstruation	Vitex	Cycle 2 Progestonic™
Fungus, lichen, Athlete's foot, candida	Black Walnut	Yeast ReLeaf™
Herpes, labial or genital	Myrrh	Mouth Tonic™
Shingles, rash in	Red Clover	Dermatonic™
Shingles, pain in	Skullcap	Nervine Tonic™
Diaper rash	Pau D'Arco	Yeast ReLeaf™
Poison ivy, poison oak, contact dermatitis	Red Root	Lymphatonic™ (internally) Ivy Itch ReLeaf™ (externally)
Hives, allergies; stop skin inflammation	Nettle	Allertonic™

Herbs for Poor Sleep

Match your "type" of insomnia or poor sleep patterns listed on the left under Symptoms to the recommended herbal extracts on the right. Unlike over-the-counter (OTC) sleeping aids, these herbs do not suppress the dream state (also known as rapid eye-movement {REM} sleep).

Symptoms	Recommended Herbs	
	Singles	*Formulas*
Insomnia from being high strung; difficult time falling asleep	Chamomile	Nervine Tonic™
Sleep problems from muscle twitches & hyper-sensitive states	Skullcap	Nervine Tonic™
Insomnia from excessive mental stimulation	Passion-flower	NervineTonic™
Major difficulty falling asleep; sleep disturbance with heart palpitation, digestive problems & headaches	Valerian	Deep Sleep®
Major difficulty staying asleep; long-standing sleep disturbances	California Poppy	Deep Sleep®
Multiple sleep disturbance symptoms		Deep Sleep® (Combines California Poppy, Valerian, Passionflower, Chamomile, & three other herbs)

California Poppy

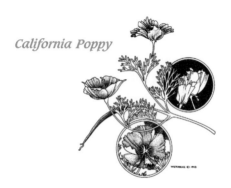

Herbs for Colds and Flu

In this table, the symptoms associated with colds and and flu are listed in chronological order in terms of what happens to the body in a typical cold or flu cycle. To prevent getting a cold or the flu in the first place, it is important to use the herbs recommended for prevention. But if you already have a cold or the flu, this table will help you choose which herbs you need to take for your specific symptoms, at the point you are in the cold cycle. For instance, Goldenseal is great for combating inflammation on the second or third day of a cold or the flu. It does not work effectively to prevent colds or the flu, as Astragalus does, or cleanse the body after a cold or the flu, as Red Root does. Effective herbal treatment of colds and flu depends on which herb is taken at what stage of the disease.

Cycle/Symptoms	Recommended Herbs	
	Singles	*Formulas*
Prevention; ongoing, way in advance of cold season	Reishi	Deep Health™
Prevention; one to two months before cold season and/or during stressful periods	Astragalus	Echinacea/ Astragalus Complex
Day one of cold/flu; body feeling achy, feverish	Echinacea	Echinacea Triple Source Plus™
Day two or three; body feeling rotten; beginning of sore throat & inflammation	Goldenseal	Goldenseal/ Echinacea Complex
Day four, five or six; cold/flu begins to infect particular area of body, i.e. mucus in the lungs	Osha	Respiratonic™
Day four, five or six; infectionis present, mucus has yellow or green color	Usnea	Phytocillin™
Day four, five or six; sore throat with laryngitis & pharyngitis	Collinsonia	Singer's Saving Grace®
Day four, five or six; cold settles in the head; runny nose, thin mucus	Ephedra &Mullein	Decongestonic™
Day four, five or six; cold settles in head; dry membranes, thick mucus	Ephedra & Yerba Mansa	Congest Free™
The really hard-to-shake or recurring cold/flu	Red Root	Lymphatonic™

Herbs for Stopping Smoking

The first thing to consider in the process of stopping smoking is your motivation. It is my clinical experience that no amount of herbs will make up for weak motivation, especially when smokers are trying to quit in order to please others. If you truly want to quit for yourself out of choice, not obligation, then your likelihood of success dramatically increases. Because nicotine addiction affects the physiology of the body in several ways, it is best to provide yourself with herbal support in a variety of areas. This table lists symptoms in six basic areas: cravings, lung congestion, nervous irritability, the weakened endocrine system, the digestive process and blood sugar imbalance. The good news is that, unlike tobacco, none of these herbs are habit forming.

Symptoms	Recommended Herbs	
	Singles	*Formulas*
Cravings; addictive alkaloids stored all over the body	Lobelia	Smoke Free Drops™
Lung congestion; choking feeling due to lung mucus	Osha	Respiratonic™
Lung congestion	Pleurisy Root	Respiratonic™
Nervous irritability; feeling as if you want to crawl out of your skin	Oat Seed	Nervine Tonic™
Nervous irritability; "chattering", busy brain	Passionflower	Nervine Tonic™
Weakened endocrine system contributes to cravings & low energy	Licorice	Adrenotonic™
Poor digestion; constipation	Gentian	Digestonic™
Blood sugar imbalance; symptoms of hypoglycemia in initial stages of stopping smoking	Woodsgrown American Ginseng	Ginseng Seven Source™
Overall herbal formula for across-the-board body support		Smoke Free Drops™ (Combines Lobelia, Oat seed, Licorice, Osha, Pleurisy Root & four other herbs)

Herbs for Allergies

Because allergies, or allergic rhinitis, can be related to a multitude of seasonal and non-seasonal irritants ranging from tree pollens to house dust, this is a difficult area to address from just one vantage point. Generally, in addition to herbal support, I urge you to take corrective measures to reduce stress in your life (sinuses and nasal membranes react to overall health and stress levels) and to improve your overall diet. Try to avoid dairy products, grains (especially wheat), sugar, alcohol and sweets, which aggravate allergies, among other things. For those who wish to go into more suggestions on how to heal allergies naturally, I recommend the following book: *Breathe Free* by Daniel Gagnon and Amadea Morningstar, published by Lotus Press, Santa Fe, New Mexico.

Symptoms	Recommended Herbs	
	Singles	*Formulas*
Prevention of hay fever sensitivity to trees, flowers & ragweeds; also during hay fever season	Nettle	Allertonic™
Prevention & support; adrenal gland support	Siberian Ginseng	Adrenotonic™
Liver support to help process inflammation that is clogging the body	Barberry	Liver Tonic™
Hay fever symptoms; sinus pain; thin mucus; lots of fluids!	Ephedra & Mullein	Decongestonic™
Hay fever symptoms; thick mucus; congestion; nothing is moving!	Ephedra & Yerba Mansa	Congest Free™
Asthma related to sensitivity to pollens	Ephedra	Congest Free™

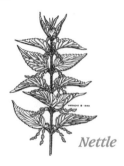

Nettle

Herbs for Digestive Problems

As stated in my discussion of the **Ten Elements of Good Health** (Chapter 1), it is extremely important for you to attend to the quality of your diet on a daily basis. However, if you are experiencing digestive problems, there are many herbs that are very effective aids to digestive system functions. Remember to practice good dietary habits and support your herbal treatments by drinking plenty of water (64 ounces a day).

Symptoms	Recommended Herbs	
	Singles	*Formulas*
Dry mouth; coated teeth & tongue in the morning	Cayenne	Digestonic™
Lack of stomach digestive enzymes, creating poor digestion; bloating after eating; indigestion	Gentian	Digestonic™
Stomach gas; bloating & burning sensation	Chamomile	Stomach Tonic™
Stomach or intestinal cramping with possible diarrhea	Cramp Bark	Cramp ReLeaf™
Poor fat absorption; oily stools; dry skin due to lack of liver bile secretion	Barberry	Liver Tonic™
Diarrhea	Bayberry	Montezuma's ReLeaf™
Candida symptoms; dermatitis; diarrhea, flatulence & "sick all over" feeling	Pau D'Arco	Yeast ReLeaf™
Sea sickness; motion sickness; nausea (even from chemotherapy or vertigo)	Ginger	

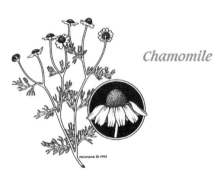

Chamomile

Herbs for Women's Reproductive System Problems

Among the various people seeking alternative therapies, women are emerging as a major force in support of herbal medicine. This support is due, in large part, to the fact that herbs offer a more harmonious and gentler way of working with the body than drugs. Herbs answer women's need to find safer, less intrusive and less disruptive treatments for female reproductive system issues. This table groups recommended herbs into four categories-herbs for menstrual distress, cycle balancing, menopause and sexual encounter-related infections.

Symptoms	Recommended Herbs	
	Singles	*Formulas*
Menstrual cramps, sharp	Cramp Bark	Cramp ReLeaf™
Menstrual congestion, dull pain down the leg	Black Cohosh and/or Blue Cohosh	Monthly ReLeaf™
Menstrual cramps, sharp; pain in muscles	Meadowsweet	Herbaprofen™
Delayed menstruation due to travel, cold, stress	Pennyroyal	
PMS symptoms; water retention; mood swings	Vitex & Dandelion	PMS ReLeaf™ Progestonic™ Cycle 2
Cycle imbalance; lack of menstruation after getting off the pill	Dong Quai & Vitex	Alternate Cycle 1 Estrotonic™ & Cycle 2 Progestonic™
Cycle imbalance; breast, ovarian, uterine cysts	Red Root	Lymphatonic™
Cycle imbalance; estrogen enhancer; day 1 of menses to day 14	Black Cohosh Dong Quai	Cycle 1 Estrotonic™
Cycle imbalance; progesterone enhancer: day 15 of cycle to day 28	Vitex	Cycle 2 Progestonic™
Menopausal symptoms	Black Cohosh, Dong Quai or Vitex	Menopautonic™
Urinary tract infection after sex	Uva Ursi	Cran-Bladder ReLeaf™
Discomfort from herpes outbreak; lesions	Echinacea	Passion Potion™

Chapter 7:

Herbal Directory

Notes on this Herbal Directory:

This section lists single extracts and formulas in alphabetical order. To find the herbs that are best suited for your health issues, you can read the description of each herb in this section. Or better yet, you can start with the **Health Condition Index**, which recommends the best herbal extracts for conditions ranging from Abdominal Pain to Yeast Infection, and then refer back to this section to look up the specific herbs you need.

Note that when an herb is designated as a "fresh herb," it means the herb has not been dried. Also, for all formulas, ingredients are listed in descending order of content. Please heed all dosage recommendations and note contraindications, possible side effects and/or warnings when applicable.

Acnetonic™ (Burdock/Violet Complex). Specific for acne that occurs in adolescence or young adulthood. Also helpful for women who experience flare-ups of acne during hormonal shifts of their menstrual cycle or during ingestion of oral contraceptives.
Ingredients: Burdock, Echinacea, Dong Quai, Sarsaparilla, Violet leaves, Oregon Grape, Licorice, Dandelion root, Yellow Dock, Red Clover, Cultivated American Ginseng, Kelp.
Dose: Take 20 drops three times a day for one month. Then take Dermatonic™ at the same dosage for the following month. Continue alternating Dermatonic™ and Acnetonic™ every other month.
Contraindications: Not in pregnancy.

Adrenotonic™ (Black Currant/Licorice Complex). Superb adrenal gland tonic. Ideal formula to take after cortico-steroidal therapy. For any illnesses that are aggravated during stressful periods, such as asthma, chronic fatigue immuno-dysfuntion syndrome

(CFIDS), hypoglycemia or allergies of all kinds. Prevents excessive response to everyday stress. A great female adaptogen as it will not disturb the menstrual cycle.

Ingredients: Black Currant leaves, Astragalus, Licorice, Siberian Ginseng, Cultivated American Ginseng, Schisandra, Sarsaparilla, Fo-ti.

Dose: Take 25 drops or one softgel twice a day. Take for at least 100 days to achieve best results.

Contraindications: Not in pregnancy.

Alfalfa (*Medicago sativa*, fresh herb). High in chlorophyll. Excellent support in arthritis, rheumatism, colitis, ulcers, and anemia. A supportive herb to use when taking sulfa or antibiotic drugs or when fasting.

Dose: Take 15-30 drops up to four times a day.

Allertonic™ (Stinging Nettle/Eyebright Complex). A formula used in cases of allergies that manifest as eczema, hay fever, hives, asthma, skin rash, sinusitis, headaches, allergic rhinitis, chronic bronchitis, itchy eyes, sneezing, inflammation of the mouth, stomach and/or intestines, diarrhea and, in some cases, arthritis. Prevents the release of inflammatory substances and reduces excessive body defense reactions.

Ingredients: Fresh Stinging Nettle, Licorice, Eyebright, Horehound, Osha, Horsetail, Mullein, Elecampane, Plantain.

Dose: Take 20-40 drops or one softgel three to five times a day. This formula may be slow acting for some individuals. Take for a minimum of two weeks. If results are positive, continue for three to six months.

Arnica (*Arnica spp.*, fresh plant). FOR EXTERNAL USE ONLY. A first aid liniment for muscular soreness and pain from sprains, bruises, strains, over-exertion; rheumatic pain, phlebitis or arthritis. Excellent for the sore "weekend warrior."

Use: Apply every few hours; wash hands after applying.

Contraindications: Do not use on broken skin and open wounds.

Side effects: May cause skin rash (allergic dermatitis) in sensitive persons, or with prolonged use.

Warning: FOR EXTERNAL USE ONLY. If the skin becomes irritated, cease use.

Arthrotonic™ (Devil's Claw/Yucca Complex). Useful in reducing pain, inflammation, swelling, and tenderness of joints and muscles. Offers relief in arthritis, rheumatoid arthritis, myositis, fibromyalgia, irritable bowel syndrome, gout, or joint inflammation of synovial membranes (those covering the joints) and joint stiffness. Increases excretion and neutralization of uric acid and other waste products that initiate and prolong inflammation.

Ingredients: Devil's Claw, Burdock, Alfalfa, Black Cohosh, Licorice, Yucca, Echinacea, Pipsissewa, Wild Indigo, Horsetail.

Dose: Take 15-25 drops or one softgel three times a day. Take for three weeks and stop for one week. Repeat cycle.

Contraindications: Not in pregnancy.

Ashwagandha (*Withania somnifera*, dried root). A good preventative herb. Increases stress endurance and prevents stress-induced stomach ulcers. Anti-inflammatory action makes it useful in rheumatoid and osteoarthritis. Good adjunct in cancer treatment, preventing weight loss and stimulating the immune system.

Dose: Take 20-30 drops three times a day. Take for 100 days or more for best results.

Contraindications: Not in pregnancy. Not for use with barbiturates.

Warning: May potentiate the effects of barbiturates.

Astragalus (*Astragalus membranaceus* [Huang Qi], dried root slice). One of the best preventative herbs available. Deep immune system tonic. Improves adrenal gland function. Useful for fatigue, frequent colds, or chronic non-healing sores. Increases production of interferon and increases resistance to viral infections.

Dose: Take 15-30 drops twice a day. Take for 100 days or more to achieve best results.

Barberry (*Berberis vulgaris*, dried root). As a bitter tonic, helps resolve indigestion and poor appetite. It improves nutrition by stimulating digestion, absorption and assimilation. Helpful for acne, psoriasis, herpes flare-ups and eczema, especially when these conditions are accompanied by constipation. Improves liver function. Also very useful in parasitic infection, especially giardia.

Dose: *As a bitter tonic, take 5 drops ten minutes before each meal. For other uses, take 10-20 drops three times a day.*

Contraindications: *Not in pregnancy.*

Bayberry (*Myrica cerifera*, dried root bark). For long term inflammation of mouth, for bleeding gums, sore throat and stomach. For diarrhea from stress, excess food; for colitis or dysentery.

Dose: *Take 15-25 drops three times a day. For bleeding gums or sore throat, dilute, then gargle and swallow.*

Bionic Tonic™ (Red Ginseng/Fo-ti Complex). Helps you stay awake, alert and mentally clear. Useful when driving, studying, doing a task over and over, or when you need to be alert, bushy-tailed and fully alive. Great as a mid-morning or mid-afternoon pick-me-up. Contains no caffeine or Ephedra (Ma Huang).

Ingredients: *Chinese Kirin Red Ginseng, Fo-ti, Gotu Kola, Siberian Ginseng, Damiana, Cultivated American Ginseng, Licorice, Prickly Ash berry, Peppermint, Ginger, Cayenne*

Dose: *Take 15-30 drops mid-morning, mid-afternoon, or other times as a pick-me-up.*

Contraindications: *Not in pregnancy.*

Side effects: *May cause insomnia.*

Black Cohosh (*Cimicifuga racemosa*, dried root). For dull aching pains without acute inflammation in joints, muscles or uterus. For weak, irregular uterine contractions during labor or for after-birth pains. Useful for menopausal women experiencing hot flashes and depression.

Dose: *Take 10-20 drops every four hours.*

Contraindications: *Not during the first seven months of pregnancy. Do not use while breast-feeding.*

Side effects: *Excessive use may cause occasional gastrointestinal discomfort, mild frontal headache, dizziness, impaired vision, vertigo, nausea, vomiting, and/or impaired circulation.*

Black Walnut (*Juglans nigra*, fresh "green" hull). For eczema, acne, lichen, candida, intestinal distress, diarrhea, chronic scaly skin diseases and

inflammation of the mouth, throat and stomach.
Dose: Take 10-20 drops up to three times a day. Not for long term use. **Externally:** *As a wash, one teaspoon of the extract in half a cup of boiled water. Apply when water cools.*
Warning: *Not for prolonged use.*

Blueberry (*Vaccinium spp.*, fresh leaf). Useful for adult onset diabetes, the type that can be controlled by diet. Lowers elevated blood sugar level. Increases uric acid elimination and relieves gout. Stops diarrhea, especially in children.
Dose: Take 20-30 drops after meals.
Warning: *Not useful in insulin-dependent diabetes.*

Blue Cohosh (*Caulophyllum thalictroides*, dried root). Use for menstrual cramps when dull pains extend to buttocks and back of legs. Facilitates childbirth when delay in labor is due to weakness, fatigue or lack of uterine power.
Dose: Take 5-15 drops up to four times a day.
Contraindications: *Not during the first seven months of pregnancy.*
Side effects: *May cause mid-cycle spotting and cramping in sensitive women.*

Burdock (*Arctium lappa*, Autumn-gathered dried root). Effective in dry and scaly eczema, psoriasis, acne, dandruff and boils. Stimulates digestive juices and bile secretion. In gout, stimulates excretion of urea and uric acid.
Dose: Take 15-25 drops three times a day for an extended period of time (three to four months).

Calendula (*Calendula officinalis*, fresh flower). **Internally:** For inflammation of the mouth and peptic ulcers. **Externally:** For healing skin burns or inflammation, abrasions, pressure ulcers (i.e., bed sores), and impetigo (also see Usnea).
Dose: Take 10-15 drops up to four times a day.
Externally: *Dilute with water and apply.*

California Poppy (*Eschscholzia californica*, fresh flowering plant). Specific for people who have difficulty falling asleep or who wake up during the night or too early in the morning. Permits deep sound sleep. Great for sleepless, frenetic children, or for children who sleep so soundly that they wet the bed.

Dose: *Take 20-40 drops one hour before sleep and again just before bedtime. For bed wetting, in children over five years old, use with Horsetail, 10 drops of each twice a day.*
Contraindications: *Not in pregnancy. Not for use with MAO-inhibitors.*
Warning: *May potentiate the effects of MAO-inhibitors.*

Cardiotonic™ (Hawthorn/Motherwort Complex). Formula for heart irregularities with rapid heart beat episodes or weakness of heart muscle. Specific support for angina, as it greatly improves the blood flow to the heart muscle. Offers excellent support in heart disease.
Ingredients: *Hawthorn flowers, leaves and berries, Motherwort, Bugleweed, Ginkgo, Passionflower, Cultivated American Ginseng, Siberian Ginseng, Rosemary.*
Dose: *Take 15-25 drops three times a day for one month, then twice a day for an unlimited period of time.*
Contraindications: *Not in pregnancy.*
Warning: *Not useful for damaged heart where the damage is termed organic. Works best for functional heart problems (i.e., angina).*

Catnip (*Nepeta cataria*, fresh pre-flowering herb). Taken hot, stimulates sweating in colds and flu, and breaks up fevers. Taken cold, eases stomach and intestinal cramps in adults and especially in children. Eases insomnia caused by muscle tension.
Dose: *Take 20-30 drops up to five times a day.*
Contraindications: *Not in pregnancy.*

Cat's Claw (*Uncaria tomentosa* [Uña de Gato], dried tree bark). Europeans report positive clinical use with AZT in treating AIDS. Genital herpes and herpes zoster both respond favorably to its use. Also helpful for diverticulitis, hemorrhoids, colitis, leaky bowel syndrome, fistulas, peptic ulcers, gastritis, gastric ulcers, candidiasis, and Crohn's disease. Cat's Claw helps to curb parasites and dysentery. Found useful in arthritis, bursitis, and rheumatism.
Dose: *Take 20-40 drops three to five times a day.*

Cayenne (*Capsicum annuum*, dried fruit). In viral infections, cools dry, hot mucous membranes. Small amounts increase secretions; useful in case of dry mouth and a lack of digestive secretions due to nervousness, alcohol abuse, prescription drugs and old age. Stimulates circulation.

Dose: Take 5-10 drops in warm water.

Contraindications: *Do not use on broken skin or near eyes.*

Side effects: *May cause stomach or intestinal irritation.*

Warning: *If the skin becomes irritated, cease use*

Chamomile (*Matricaria recutita*, whole fresh flower). **Internally:** Useful for anxiety, insomnia, indigestion, flatulence, gastritis, stomach ulcers, gingivitis, gastro-enteritis, colitis and menstrual related migraines. **Externally:** Reduces inflammation and speeds up healing of wounds.

Dose: For adults, take 20-50 drops up to four times a day. For babies, give 1-2 drops, diluted in a liquid, up to three times a day.

Note: *Safe for babies two months and older.*

Chaparral (*Larrea tridentata*, dried leaf). Helpful in autoimmune and allergic disorders. For people who have been in long-term contact with chemicals, metals or aromatic hydrocarbons, such as solvents, paints and thinners. Also for poor digestion and assimilation of dietary fats.

Dose: Take 20 drops up to three times a day.

Contraindications: *Not in pregnancy. Not in pre-existing kidney disease or liver conditions such as hepatitis or cirrhosis.*

Warning: *Discontinue use if nausea, fever, fatigue or jaundice (e.g. dark or yellow discoloration of the eyes) should occur.*

Chaste Tree (see Vitex)

Chickweed (*Stellaria media*, fresh herb). **Internally:** Useful as a diuretic for PMS water retention and for overly acidic urine from excessive meat eating or steroid intake. **Externally:** Use as a rub for arthritis, rheumatism, sprains or gout.

Dose: Take 15-25 drops three times a day.

Externally: *Dilute with water and apply.*

Chlorophyll Concentrate™ (extracted from English Stinging Nettles). Use for low red blood cell count, fatigue, shortness of breath, high altitude sickness, or heavy menstrual flow. Intestinal deodorizer.

Dose: Each 36-drop dose delivers 100 milligrams of Chlorophyll Concentrate™. Take 20-35 drops (before meals) three times a day.

Side effects: Dark green stools may occur.

Cholesterotonic™ (Siberian Ginseng/Devil's Claw Complex). For elevated cholesterol and/or triglyceride levels, especially during periods of physical or emotional stress. Helps to increase high density lipoproteins (HDL, the good cholesterol) and decrease low density lipoproteins (LDL, the bad cholesterol). Also helpful when these elevations are due to excessive alcohol and/or fat intake.

Ingredients: Siberian Ginseng, Devil's Claw, Cultivated American Ginseng, Greater Celandine, Fo-ti, Shepherd's Purse, Couchgrass, Prickly Ash.

Dose: Take 15-20 drops or one softgel three times a day after meals.

Contraindications: Not in pregnancy.

Collinsonia (*Collinsonia canadensis*, Autumn-gathered fresh root). Useful for throat irritation from intensive talking, singing or shouting, as in pharyngitis and laryngitis. Also, for hemorrhoids and varicosities due to poor venous blood circulation with a sense of constriction, rectal pain and bladder irritation with painful urination.

Dose: Take 30-40 drops up to four times a day. For irritation of throat, dilute, then gargle and swallow.

Congest Free™ (Ephedra [Ma Huang]/Yerba Mansa Complex). For sinus congestion with hot dry membranes, headache, pain, pressure and heaviness in the sinuses, low fever, blocked ears, earache and even bleeding nose from dryness. Take if mucus is thick, if it is difficult to blow your nose and if it feels like your head is in a vice-like grip. Good to use when you are congested and must travel by plane.

Ingredients: Ephedra [Ma Huang], Yerba Mansa, Cubeb berries, Eyebright, Osha, Cayenne.

Dose: For general usage, take 15-25 drops every four hours. If taken specifically for travel via plane, take 60-80 drops one hour and a half prior to landing.

Contraindications: Not in pregnancy or while breast-feeding. Not in anorexia, bulimia, or glaucoma.

Side effects: May cause insomnia, nervousness, tremor, loss of appetite, nausea or high blood pressure.
Warning: Seek advice from a health care practitioner prior to use if you have high blood pressure, heart or thyroid disease, diabetes, difficulty in urination due to prostate enlargement; or if taking an MAO inhibitor. Reduce or discontinue use if nervousness, tremor, sleeplessness, loss of appetite, nausea, or high blood pressure occur. Do not take for more than six weeks in succession.

Cramp Bark (*Viburnum opulus*, dried bark and root bark). Calms painful menstruation with stabbing-like pains, severe discomfort and abundant bleeding. Calms the stomach, intestines, heart and nervous system. Useful for morning sickness and for threatened miscarriage in the last trimester.
Dose: Take 20-60 drops up to every two hours if needed.

Cramp ReLeaf™ (Black Haw/Cramp Bark Complex). Relieves sharp, strong menstrual cramps occurring prior to or during menstruation. Calms diarrhea and upset stomach that accompany menstruation. Improves ovarian and uterine circulation, soothes the pelvic muscles and promotes toning of the entire birthing organ. Reduces morning sickness and controls after-birth pains. In combination with Shepherd's Purse, it prevents postpartum hemorrhage.
Ingredients: Black Haw, Cramp Bark, Beth Root, Cloves, Cinnamon, Wild Yam, Cardamom, Orange peel.
Dose: Take 40-100 drops, or one-half to one teaspoon in warm water, every three or four hours.

Cran-Bladder ReLeaf™ (Cranberry/Uva Ursi Complex). Prevents and stops recurring urinary tract infection (UTI), especially in females, in two ways: 1) prevents bacteria from sticking to the walls of the bladder, and 2) oils from the herbs help deactivate and destroy the bacteria that are present in the bladder, urethra, and ureters. Stimulates the immune system of the urinary tract, acidifies the urine and tones the urinary system. Specific to prevent infection occurring after intercourse.

Ingredients: *Cranberry, Uva Ursi, Echinacea, Stinging Nettles, Buchu, Horsetail, Pipsissewa, Yarrow, Meadowsweet, Licorice, Stevia.*

Dose: *For acute symptoms, take 20 drops every hour or two. For chronic conditions, take 30 drops twice a day for an unlimited amount of time as a preventative.*

Contraindications: *Not in pregnancy.*

Side effects: *Peculiar urine smell and color may occur.*

Cycle 1 Estrotonic™ Support for days 1-14
Cycle 2 Progestonic™ Support for days 15-28

These combinations were formulated to be used in tandem: for regulating menstrual cycles for women who are getting off oral contraceptives or who have erratic menstrual cycles due to a variety of interruptions such as breast feeding, physical reactions to travel, trauma, etc.; for women who are having difficulty conceiving; for women who have excessively long or short menstrual cycles. Three to six months of alternating Cycle 1 Estrotonic™ and Cycle 2 Progestonic™ will re-establish a normal and balanced cycle. These formulas work together over the course of the 28-day menstrual cycle and should be taken as follows:

Cycle 1 Estrotonic™ Day 1-14 Support (Black Cohosh/ Dong Quai Complex). This formula specifically balances estrogen levels in order to reestablish proper timing of the menstrual cycle and to facilitate ovulation.

Ingredients: *Black Cohosh, Dong Quai, Shatavari, False Unicorn, Partridge berry, Licorice, Cultivated American Ginseng, Stevia.*

Dose: *Take 30 drops twice a day for the first half of the menstrual cycle. Begin taking from the first day of menstruation to the fourteenth day (ovulation). On the fifteenth day, switch to Cycle 2 Progestonic™.*

Contraindications: *Not in pregnancy.*

Cycle 2 Progestonic™ Day 15-28 Support (Vitex/Wild Yam Complex). This formula increases the production of progesterone in balance with estrogen levels established in the first half of the menstrual cycle. Aids conception, because increased progesterone promotes proper implantation of the fertilized egg. Can be taken specifically for PMS symptoms without alternating with Cycle 1 Estrotonic™; helps relieve water retention, swollen and tender breasts, lower backache, cramping, fatigue, irritability, insomnia, depression, difficulty in concentrating, panic attacks, anxiety, mood swings, crying, physical and emotional tension, low blood sugar, low sex drive, headaches and migraines.

Ingredients: Vitex, Wild Yam, Dandelion, Reishi, Blue Cohosh, Chickweed, Shatavari, Black Haw, Cinnamon, Orange peel.

Dose: Take 30 drops twice a day for the second half of the menstrual cycle. Begin taking on the fifteenth day of the menstrual cycle and continue until the first day of next menstruation. Then switch to Cycle 1 Estrotonic™. Keep alternating Cycle 1 Estrotonic™ and Cycle 2 Progestonic™ for three to six months to achieve best results. If used specifically for PMS symptoms rather than for regulation of menstrual cycle, begin taking 30 drops up to twice a day, 8-10 days prior to onset of menstruation.

Contraindications: Not in pregnancy.

Damiana (*Turnera spp.*, dried leaf). Useful in anxiety and depression. Use for irritation of urinary passages (urethra or bladder) from emotional stress, sexual stress, or stress due to traveling. For delayed menstruation in young girls. Has a reputation as an aphrodisiac.

Dose: Take 20-40 drops in warm water three times a day.

Dandelion (*Taraxacum officinale*, fresh Autumn-gathered root, leaf and flower). For poor bile secretion, poor appetite and digestive function, constipation from lack of bile, rheumatic conditions, eczema, chronic skin eruptions, or psoriasis aggravated by emotional stress and/or fatty foods. As a potassium-rich diuretic, helpful for water retention due to heart problems, PMS or heat sickness.

Dose: Take 20-40 drops three or four times a day.

Contraindications: Not for use where there is blockage of the bile ducts, acute gallbladder inflammation, and intestinal blockage.

Decongestonic™ (Ephedra [Ma Huang]/Mullein Complex). For head colds with runny nose, teary, itchy eyes, sneezing and postnasal drip. Use when there is a lot of thin moving clear mucus present. Excellent for hay fever, sinus inflammation, allergy-induced asthma or bronchitis. Dries out sinuses and respiratory passages.

Ingredients: *Ephedra [Ma Huang], Mormon Tea, Mullein, Yerba Santa, Eyebright, Cubeb.*

Dose: *Take 15-30 drops every four hours.*

Contraindications: *Not in pregnancy or while breast-feeding. Not in anorexia, bulimia, or glaucoma.*

Side effects: *May cause insomnia, nervousness, tremor, loss of appetite, nausea or high blood pressure.*

Warning: *Seek advice from a health care practitioner prior to use if you have high blood pressure, heart or thyroid disease, diabetes, difficulty in urination due to prostate enlargement; or if taking an MAO inhibitor. Reduce or discontinue use if nervousness, tremor, sleeplessness, loss of appetite, nausea, or high blood pressure occur. Do not take for more than six weeks in succession.*

Deep Chi Builder™ (see **Deep Health™**)

Deep Health™ (formerly called **Deep Chi Builder™**) (Reishi/Shiitake Complex). A daily multi-herbal formula. High quality deep immune system toner. Has anti-cancer, anti-tumor, immunostimulating, and adaptogenic properties. Protects the liver, kidneys, stomach and heart. Useful in reducing high cholesterol and high triglyceride levels. Helps relieve nervousness, anxiety, sleeplessness, dizziness, chronic hepatitis, allergies, heart disease, high blood pressure, and stomach and intestinal ulcers, as well as chronic respiratory problems such as asthma, emphysema and bronchitis. Prevents blood clot formation and stabilizes blood sugar problems. Excellent support for HIV, ARC, and AIDS treatment, and as a cancer preventative or with orthodox cancer therapy. Helps to rebuild the body after long, serious or debilitating diseases. Helps prevent antibiotic-resistant bacterial infections.

Ingredients: *Reishi mushroom, Shiitake mushroom, California Spikenard, Astragalus, Maitake*

mushroom, Ashwagandha, Siberian Ginseng, Schisandra, Cordyceps, Ginger.
Dose: *Take 20 to 30 drops or one softgel twice a day as a daily multi-herbal formula.*

Deep Sleep® (California Poppy/Valerian Complex). Specific for inability to fall asleep, waking up during the night, or waking up too early in the morning. For insomnia resulting from depression, for waking up groggy or tired, as well as for fitful and/or agitated sleep. For sleep problems accompanied by cramps or pain. For insomnia while weaning from drugs, alcohol or cigarettes. Also for inability to fall asleep from tiredness. Helps to reeducate the brain sleep center.
Ingredients: *California Poppy, Valerian, Passionflower, Chamomile, Lemon Balm, Oat seed, Orange peel.*
Dose: *Take 30-60 drops or one softgel one hour before bedtime and again at bedtime. Best results are achieved by the second or third night.*

Deprezac™ (St. John's Wort/Lemon Balm Complex). Formula specific for mild to medium depression. Possesses sedative and anti-depressant effects. Decreases feelings of anxiety, tension, fatigue, irritability, depression, insomnia, agitation, loss of appetite, loss of interest and excessive sleeping. Useful for seasonal affective disorder (SAD).
Ingredients: *St. John's Wort, Lemon Balm, Kola nut, Oat seed, Peppermint, Valerian, Siberian Ginseng, Rosemary, Damiana, Stevia.*
Dose: *Take 30 drops three times a day for three weeks, then 30 drops twice a day for at least six months.*
Warning: *Not effective for bi-polar syndrome and/or for any other severe pathological depressive states.*

Dermatonic™ (Red Clover/Burdock Complex). Helpful for cases of eczema, psoriasis, contact dermatitis. Eases itching, oozing, thickening or scaling of the skin. Speeds up healing and development of smooth, pliable skin. Use with Allertonic™ if skin problem is due to allergic reaction. For acne, alternate with Acnetonic™.
Ingredients: *Red Clover, Burdock, Pleurisy Root, Dandelion, Oregon Grape, Echinacea, Gotu Kola, Butternut, Devil's Club, Blue Flag.*

Dose: *Take 20-30 drops three times a day.*
Contraindications: *Not in pregnancy.*

Devil's Claw (*Harpagophytum procumbens*, dried secondary tuber). Safe anti-inflammatory for arthritis, rheumatism, gout, joint inflammation, gall bladder problems with pancreatic distress, and for elevated cholesterol and uric acid blood levels.
Dose: *Take 30 drops three times a day. Take for three weeks and stop for one week. Repeat cycle.*
Contraindications: *Not in gastric and duodenal ulcers.*

Digestonic™ (Gentian/Angelica Complex). Sure acting tonic for the stomach. Use for poor appetite, acid indigestion, and poor stomach or intestinal function. Stimulates breakdown of food and assimilation of nutrients. Use in anemia, nausea, vomiting or diarrhea, and recurring canker or mouth sores (aphtous stomatitis).
Ingredients: *Gentian, Quassia, Angelica, Oregon Grape, Bayberry, Cardamom.*
Dose: *Take 5-15 drops, ten to twenty minutes before meals. Use Stomach Tonic™ between meals.*
Contraindications: *Not in pregnancy.*

Dong Quai (*Angelica sinensis* [Dang Qui], cured root slice). In deficient estrogen or testosterone secretion, it increases cellular uptake of these hormones in uterine, vaginal, ovarian or prostatic disorders. For menopausal distress. For PMS with dull aching pain before or during menstruation.
Dose: *Take 10-15 drops up to three times a day.*
Contraindications: *Not in pregnancy. Not during acute inflammation of above mentioned tissues.*

Echinacea (*Echinacea angustifolia*, dried root). A must in the beginning stages of a cold or flu. Increases production, maturation and aggressiveness of white blood cells against intruders. Great on swollen areas due to bee, wasp, gnat and mosquito bites. Helps reduce swelling and stimulates repair of tendons, ligaments and muscle sheaths. Excellent for tendonitis, bursitis, tennis elbow, skier's knee and jogger's ankle. Prevents or slows down bacterial and viral infections by strengthening connective tissues. Gets rid of dead microbes, dead cells and other waste products by stimulating lymphatic drainage.

Dose: *For acute symptoms, take 10-40 drops every hour. If chronic, take 20-40 drops up to four times a day.*

Echinacea/Astragalus Complex A deep immune system activator. Best tonic to use during the change of seasons to support and boost the immune system. Helps prevent colds and flu by increasing interferon production (interferon alerts the body at the first sign of an infection and prepares the body to deal with invaders). Use to build the immune system before stressful times or while traveling. Helps prevent recurring middle ear infections (otitis media) in children. Also for acute tonsillitis, genital or oral herpes, upper respiratory tract infection. For chronic yeast infection, thrush and contact dermatitis.

Ingredients: *Fresh Echinacea angustifolia root and herb, fresh and dried Echinacea purpurea root, dried Echinacea angustifolia root, Astragalus, Osha, Echinacea purpurea seed, Calendula.*

Dose: *As a tonic, take 20 drops or one softgel twice a day for 30 days. For acute symptoms, take 20 drops or one softgel every hour. If chronic, take 15-20 drops or one softgel three or four times a day.*

Echinacea/Elderberry Complex Excellent anti-bacterial or antiviral agent for first day of a cold or flu. This formula combines good tasting Elderberry with the time-proven properties of Echinacea. Elderberry aids in deactivating the influenza virus while Echinacea activates the immune system. For more information on the properties of each herb see the listing under both Echinacea and Elderberry.

Ingredients: *Dried Echinacea angustifolia root, fresh Elderberry.*

Dose: *In acute situations, take 40 drops every hour. As a preventative, take 30 drops twice a day.*

Echinacea Triple Source™ A complete spectrum, full-potency Echinacea formula rooted in native North American traditional medicine, and in cutting edge European phytopharmaceutical research. As a first line immune system activator, it is ideal for the initial stages of colds and at the beginning of a general infection. Stimulates production, maturation, mobilization and aggressiveness of white blood cells and other body defenses against intruders. Prevents or slows down bacterial and viral infections by strengthening the connective tissues. Helps boost the immune system prior to cold and flu season. Helps reduce swelling and stimulates repair in tendonitis, bursitis, tennis elbow and other sports injuries. Also for tonsillitis, herpes, respiratory system infection, candida, thrush and contact dermatitis.

Ingredients: Fresh and dry Echinacea root from two species (angustifolia and purpurea), fresh Echinacea angustifolia and purpurea herb, dried Echinacea pallida root, Echinacea purpurea seed.

Dose: In acute situations, take 40 drops or one softgel every hour. As a preventative, take 30 drops or one softgel twice a day.

Echinacea Triple Source Plus™ (Echinacea w/ Olive leaf, Elderberry and Spilanthes). A complete spectrum full potency Echinacea formula with the added benefits of Olive leaf, Elderberry and Spilanthes. Olive leaf has been shown to be effective against dozens of different viruses. It lessens the symptoms of herpes infections. Elderberry is helpful in deactivating the influenza virus. Spilanthes further supports the benefits of Echinacea by stimulating the immune system.

Ingredients: An Echinacea blend (fresh Echinacea angustifolia and purpurea root, dried Echinacea angustifolia and pallida roots, fresh Echinacea angustifolia and purpurea flowering herb juice, dried Echinacea purpurea mature seeds), Olive leaf, fresh Elderberry, fresh Spilanthes.

Dose:If symptoms are acute, take 20-30 drops or one softgel every hour. If chronic, take 20-40 drops or one softgel three times a day.

Elderberry (*Sambucus nigra*, fresh berry). New research indicates it is helpful in deactivating the influenza virus. Taken in the early stages of flu, it prevents symptoms from taking hold. Used traditionally as a spring cleanser. Helps get rid of excess mucus production.

Dose: Take 40 drops every four hours at the first sign of the flu.

Ephedra (*Ephedra sinica* [Ma Huang], dried twig). For hay fever, head colds, sinus congestion or allergy-induced asthma.

....

Dose: *Take 20 drops every four hours.*
Contraindications: *Not in pregnancy or while breast-feeding. Not in anorexia, bulimia, or glaucoma.*
Side effects: *May cause insomnia, nervousness, tremor, loss of appetite, nausea or high blood pressure.*
Warning: *Seek advice from a health care practitioner prior to use if you have high blood pressure, heart or thyroid disease, diabetes, difficulty in urination due to prostate enlargement; or if taking an MAO inhibitor. Reduce or discontinue use if nervousness, tremor, sleeplessness, loss of appetite, nausea, or high blood pressure occur. Do not take for more than six weeks in succession.*
Note: *Ephedra (Ma Huang) should not be used as a stimulant, to "give" one energy, or for weight loss.*

Essiac Tonic (Burdock/Sheep Sorrel Complex). This formula was originally given to Canadian nurse Rene Caisse by a Chippewa Indian. Helps move the body toward a state of integration and health. Alleviates and gets rid of chronic and degenerative diseases. Boosts the immune system, cleanses and supports the liver and the blood. Useful in autoimmune disorders, allergic disorders, and chronic fatigue immuno-dysfunction syndrome (CFIDS).
Ingredients: *Burdock, Sheep Sorrel, Slippery Elm, Turkey Rhubarb.*
Dose: *If symptoms are acute, take one softgel or 40 drops in two ounces of hot water twice a day, morning and evening, on an empty stomach for 32 days. Take one week off. Repeat cycle. For prevention, take for one month twice a year. Do not eat or drink anything for at least one hour after taking Essiac Tonic™.*
Contraindications: *Not in pregnancy.*

Eyebright (*Euphrasia officinalis*, dried herb). Internally: Take for hay fever and allergies with watery eyes, sneezing, runny nose, frontal headache and stuffy sinuses. Externally: In diluted form use for rapid relief of redness and swelling in conjunctivitis or blepharitis.
Dose: Internally: *Take 20-30 drops every three hours.*
Externally: *Must dilute. Mix 20 drops in 1/4 cup hot water. Let water cool and use as a wash.*

Fennel (*Foeniculum vulgare*, dried seed). Eliminates flatulence. Very useful for babies who have gas and distressed digestive systems (i.e., diarrhea, dyspepsia, intestinal spasms). Increases milk secretion in nursing mothers.
Dose: *For adults, take 30-40 drops up to four times a day. For babies, give 1-2 drops, diluted in a liquid, up to three times a day.*
Note: *Safe for babies two months and older.*

Feverfew (*Tanacetum parthenium*, fresh and dried leaf). Use for neuralgia and for spasms of the alimentary canal (gut). Useful for migraine headaches, rheumatoid arthritis and psoriasis when taken for at least three months.
Dose: *Take 15-30 drops every day for migraine prevention or other symptoms. Can be taken for an unlimited period of time. Taking 30 drops of the extract every half-hour during attacks may stop some acute migraine headaches.*
Contraindications: *Not in pregnancy.*
Side effects: *Mouth ulceration or gastric disturbance may occur.*

Fo-ti (*Polygonum multiflorum* [Ho shou wu], dried root slice). For physical debility, high cholesterol levels, and weakness. Long-term immune system tonic.
Dose: *Take 15-30 drops three times a day. Take for 100 days to achieve best results.*
Contraindications: *Not when diarrhea is present.*

Gentian (*Gentiana lutea*, dried root). For poor appetite, acid indigestion, poor stomach or intestinal function. Stimulates digestive function after prolonged illness. For anemia or when recuperating from nausea, vomiting or diarrhea.
Dose: *Take 5-15 drops in a little water at least 10 minutes before meals.*
Contraindications: *Not when gastric and duodenal ulcers, gastric irritation, and inflammation are present.*

Ginger (*Zingiber officinale*, dried root). Relieves motion sickness, nausea (even from chemotherapy or vertigo), and vomiting better than "Dramamine®." Relieves indigestion, abdominal and menstrual cramping, dyspepsia and gastric hypoacidity. Helps with acute colds and flu.

Dose: Take 10-20 drops three times a day before meals. For motion sickness, take 30-60 drops thirty minutes before your trip. Repeat every two to four hours.

Ginkgo (*Ginkgo biloba*, fresh and dry Autumn-gathered yellowing leaf). Has a scavenging effect on free radicals. For hearing and sight disorders with poor blood flow in ears and eyes; tinnitus. Helpful for Alzheimer's disease, vertigo associated with inner ear problems; loss of memory and alertness. Helps prevent poor circulation problems in eyes, skin, and extremities when diabetes is present.

Dose: Take 20-30 drops up to four times a day. Maximum benefits are achieved when used for at least six months to one year.

Ginseng, Chinese Kirin Red (*Panax ginseng*, cured dried root). Most stimulating of the Ginsengs. For physical or emotional stress or exhaustion, mild depression, tiredness. Very helpful to older people whose appetite, energy and stamina are low, especially while recuperating from disease or surgery.

Dose: Take 5-20 drops two to three times a day.

Contraindications: *Not for use when thyroid disease, high blood pressure, hyperglycemia or insomnia are present.*

Side effects: *May cause insomnia.*

Ginseng, Cultivated American (*Panax quinquefolius*, dried root). Used for the same conditions indicated under Woodsgrown American Ginseng. The difference between Cultivated American Ginseng and Woodsgrown American Ginseng is that Cultivated American Ginseng is considered a fair quality Ginseng because it is cultivated for six to seven years; whereas Woodsgrown is cultivated for one year, transplanted in the forest and left to grow for five to six years. Chinese connoisseurs value both Ginsengs but Woodsgrown Ginseng is more prized and fetches higher prices.

Dose: Take 15-30 drops in late afternoon.

Ginseng, Korean White (*Panax ginseng*, dried root). Considered stronger than Siberian Ginseng, but weaker than Woodsgrown American Ginseng. For emotional and physical stress manifesting as elevated blood sugar (triglycerides) and blood lipids (cholesterol), exhaustion and depression. Use when recuperating from illness or surgery. An excellent adaptogen (i.e., a substance that produces a normalizing effect on the body), it increases strength, endurance, and resistance to stress or infection.

Dose: Take 15-25 drops in morning and afternoon.

Ginseng, Siberian (*Eleutherococcus senticosus*, dried root and root bark). Not a true "Panax" Ginseng as with the other Ginsengs listed here, but has very similar actions. It works more slowly than true ginseng but it can be taken for extended periods of time. As an adaptogen (i.e., a substance that produces a normalizing effect on the body), it increases strength, endurance, and resistance to stress or infection. Useful for those who have decreased resistance due to stimulant, alcohol and drug use. Also helpful for those who thrive on stress (type A personalities).

Dose: Take 20 drops three times a day.

Ginseng, Woodsgrown American (*Panax quinquefolius*, dried root). For emotional and physical stress manifesting as elevated blood sugar (triglycerides) and blood lipids (cholesterol), exhaustion and depression. Use when recuperating from illness or surgery. As an excellent adaptogen (i.e., a substance that produces a normalizing effect on the body), it increases strength, endurance, and resistance to stress or infection.

Dose: Take 15-30 drops in late afternoon.

Ginsengs Seven Source™ The ultimate Ginseng tonic. Most complete, well rounded rejuvenating product available. Excellent for emotional or physical exhaustion, as a tonic after a prolonged illness or in depression from major neurological or autoimmune disease. A great extract to help prepare for or recuperate from major stress. Best adaptogenic formula to support and enhance your well being.

Ingredients: Woodsgrown American Ginseng, Kirin Chinese Red Ginseng, Shui-Chu Chinese Red Ginseng, Korean White Ginseng, Cultivated American Ginseng, Siberian Ginseng, Wild American Ginseng.

Dose: Take 10-25 drops twice a day for at least one

....

month to achieve best results.

Goldenseal (*Hydrastis canadensis*, dried root and rhizome). Use for sub-acute or chronic mucous membrane inflammation occurring in sinusitis, hay fever, allergies, gastritis, stomach ulcers, colitis, diarrhea, sore gums and throat, or tonsillitis.
Dose: *Take 10-25 drops up to five times a day.*
Contraindications: *Not in pregnancy.*
Warning: *Use only until the inflammatory stage goes away, then discontinue use. Not for long term use. Do not exceed recommended dose.*

Goldenseal/Echinacea Complex A favorite for fighting a cold or flu. Reduces inflammation and strengthens tissues of the throat, sinuses and bronchioles. Liquefies mucus, relieves deep-seated joint, muscle and bone pains, and headaches, as well as generalized body aches and headaches. Breaks fevers and stimulates the immune system's response. Quickly eliminates waste products and helps the body regain its balance.
Ingredients: *Echinacea, Goldenseal, Licorice, Yerba Mansa, Yarrow blossom, Elder blossom, Boneset, Bayberry, Dandelion, Grindelia, Ginger, Red Root, Osha.*
Dose: *If symptoms are acute, take 20-30 drops or one softgel every hour. For other indications, take 20-30 drops or one softgel three to four times a day.*
Contraindications: *Not in pregnancy.*

Gotu Kola (*Centella asiatica*, dried herb). Enhances memory, clarity and calmness. Great support for the thyroid gland when low function contributes to emotional depression, dry skin, cold extremities, poor digestion, weight gain and/or little endurance. Use also for eczema, psoriasis and varicose veins.
Dose: *Take 20-30 drops morning and mid-afternoon.*

Hawthorn (*Crataegus spp.*, fresh flower, terminal leaf and berry). For heart irregularities with rapid heart beat episodes or weakness of heart muscle from poor blood supply. Prevents complications in many heart diseases, especially angina and congestive heart failure.
Dose: *Take 10-20 drops up to three times a day for one month, then twice a day for an unlimited period*

of time.

Contraindications: *Do not use with digitalis.*
Warning: *May potentiate the effects of digitalis,*
consult primary care practitioner prior to use with
digitalis. Not useful for damaged heart where the
damage is termed organic. Works best for functional
heart problems (i.e., angina).

HB Pressure Tonic™ (Linden/Hawthorn Complex). Helpful in cases of mild to moderately elevated blood pressure. Especially helpful when high blood pressure is due to stress or is aggravated by excessive sodium intake. Useful in either systolic or diastolic elevations.

Ingredients: *Linden flower, Mistletoe, Dandelion,*
Passionflower, Hawthorn flower, leaf and berry,
Siberian Ginseng, Yarrow, Skullcap, Prickly Ash bark.
Dose: *Take 20-40 drops two or three times a day.*
Contraindications: *Not in pregnancy.*
Side effects: *May cause low blood pressure.*
Warning: *Monitor your blood pressure to make sure*
the herbal treatment is effective for you.

Herbaprofen™ (Jamaican Dogwood/Black Cohosh Complex). A good muscular anti-spasmodic and anti-inflammatory formula. As a botanical analgesic, it helps reduce pain and spasms caused by toothaches, uterine and fallopian cramps, neuralgia, intestinal colic, gallstones and renal colics, rheumatoid arthritis, fibrositis, sore muscles, spasmodic cough, sciatica, sprained back, etc. Useful for congestive headaches. Especially beneficial when pain prevents sleep.

Ingredients: *Jamaican Dogwood, Black Cohosh,*
Wood Betony, Meadowsweet, Kava, Passionflower,
Devil's Claw, Licorice, Stevia.
Dose: *Take 20-50 drops or one softgel up to every*
three hours, or as needed.
Contraindications: *Not in pregnancy or while breast-*
feeding.

Hops (*Humulus lupulus*, dry strobile). For insomnia caused by heartburn, indigestion, restlessness and/or headaches. Calms hyper-secretion of stomach acids while toning up digestive functions. Effective against gram-positive bacteria (Staph, Strep and Pneumonococcus).

Dose: Take 10-40 drops three times a day.
Contraindications: Not during depression.
Side effects: Long term use may cause depression.

Horsetail (*Equisetum arvense*, fresh Spring-gathered herb). Stops slow oozing bleeding of all kinds. Useful for children who wet the bed. Useful with connective tissue weaknesses as may be found in kidneys, lungs and liver. High in silica. Stimulates calcium absorption. Useful in arthritis.
Dose: Take 15-30 drops up to three times a day. For bed wetting in children over five years old, use with California Poppy, 10 drops of each twice a day.
Contraindications: Not in cardiac or renal dysfunction.

Hyssop (*Hyssopus officinalis*, fresh and dry herb). For lung problems characterized by excess mucus production with difficult expectoration. Useful for coughs, bronchitis, asthma, chronic mucus, gas, and stomach irritation.
Dose: Take 10-40 drops up to four times a day.
Contraindications: Not in pregnancy.

Ivy Itch ReLeaf™ (Jewelweed/Plantain Complex). FOR EXTERNAL USE ONLY. Stimulates healing in poison ivy or poison oak dermatitis. May also be used for herpes outbreaks (mouth or genital). Offers relief in cases of insect stings and bites, as well as rashes caused by stinging nettles.
Ingredients: Jewelweed, Grindelia, Plantain, Licorice, Echinacea.
Dose: Spray liberally on affected areas every two hours. Let dry.
Warning: FOR EXTERNAL USE ONLY.

Juniper (*Juniperus communis*, dried berry). Useful as an antiseptic in sub-acute or chronic inflammation of the bladder or urethra, i.e., the kind of inflammation that has been there for a while and has not healed properly. Also for chronic arthritis, gout and rheumatism.
Dose: Take 15-30 drops three times a day.
Contraindications: Not in pregnancy. Not in acute urinary tract infection, stomach inflammation or serious kidney disease.
Side effects: May aggravate stomach or kidney inflammation.

Warning: *Do not use for more than six weeks in succession. Do not exceed recommended dose.*

Kava *(Piper methysticum,* dried root). Useful in relieving nervousness, agitation, tension, stress and anxiety. Kava is a mood elevator; it helps relax muscle tension due to stress, relieves fatigue and calms the mind. It is very useful when anxiety prevents sleep.
Dose: *Take 20-30 drops two to three times a day.*
Contraindications: *Not in pregnancy or while breast-feeding. Do not use with alcohol or barbiturates.*
Side effects: *Large amounts over an extended period of time may cause skin rash.*
Warning: *May potentiate the effects of alcohol or barbituates. Chronic situations may require long-term use. Do not exceed recommended dose. If skin rash occurs, cease use.*

Kava Cool Complex™ (Kava/Chamomile Complex). Useful for anxiety, edginess, tension, mental and physical agitation, as well as for other symptoms of nervousness and high level stress. Helps relax muscle tension due to stress. Permits sleep when insomnia is due to muscle and/or mental tension. Acts as a mood elevator; is useful in depression where there is a lot of agitation, anxiety and inability to relax.
Ingredients: *Kava, Chamomile, St. John's Wort, Oat seed, Passionflower, Hops, Skullcap, Stevia.*
Dose: *Take 15-25 drops or one softgel three to four times a day.*
Contraindications: *Not in pregnancy or while breast-feeding. Do not use with alcohol or barbiturates.*
Side effects: *Large amounts over an extended period of time may cause skin rash.*
Warning: *May potentiate the effects of alcohol or barbituates. Chronic situations may require long-term use. Do not exceed recommended dose. If skin rash occurs, cease use.*
Note: *If taken for depression, consider alternating with Deprezac™.*

Kidalin® (Catnip/Kola Complex). Specific for attention deficit disorder (ADD) also known as attention deficit hyperactivity disorder (ADHD). Reduces aggressiveness, focuses and relaxes the mind, rebuilds the nervous system and calms the hyperkinetic behavior in those with ADHD. Lessens symptoms such as short attention span, jitteriness, restlessness, difficulty concentrating, constant shifting and fretting, difficulty completing assigned tasks, excessive running, climbing and talking. Also helpful if symptoms manifest as an inability to focus and pay attention without symptoms of overactivity or impulsivity.

Ingredients: *Catnip, Damiana, Kola nut, Lavender, Chamomile, Periwinkle, Lemon Balm, Licorice, Oat seed. Comes in natural cherry, orange or adult formulas.*

Dose: *Syrup for children five to nine years old, take one half teaspoon every four hours. Syrup for children ten years old and older, take one teaspoon twice a day. Extract for adults; take 20-40 drops two to three times a day.*

Contraindications: *Not in pregnancy.*

Kidney Tonic™ (Dandelion/Uva Ursi Complex). For non-specific inflammation of the kidneys or bladder, lower back pain, water retention in PMS or from changes in heat or humidity. Use in low grade bacterial infection of the urethra or bladder and irritation of the urethra after sex. Useful for frequent, urgent, burning or painful urination, lower back pain, pain in the pubic area, the tendency to urinate excessively at night, changes in the color of the urine, and decreases in the amount of the urine. Used over a period of time, it will strengthen the urinary system.

Ingredients: *Dandelion leaf, Saw Palmetto, Parsley root, Couchgrass, Boldo, Buchu, Juniper, Uva Ursi, Pipsissewa, Cubeb.*

Dose: *For acute situations take 20-30 drops or one softgel every four hours.*

Contraindications: *Not in pregnancy.*

Side effects: *Peculiar urine smell and color may occur.*

Licorice (*Glycyrrhiza glabra*, dried root). Effective adrenal gland support. For gastric ulcers, bronchial spasms, sore throats, painful menstruation, arthritis or herpes. Offers support in AIDS as research suggests it may inhibit the virus. Also has mild anti-inflammatory, antihistaminic and laxative properties.

Dose: *Take 20-30 drops up to three times a day.*

Contraindications: *Not in pregnancy or while breast-feeding and in hypokalemia (low blood potassium level), or when high blood pressure from sodium retention is present.*

Side effects: *Large amounts over an extended period of time may cause high blood pressure, water retention, headache, and vertigo.*

Warning: *May potentiate potassium depletion of thiazide diuretics, stimulant laxatives, cardiac glycosides or cortisol. Prolonged use is not recommended.*

Liver Tonic™ (Milk Thistle/Oregon Grape Complex). Protects and repairs the liver. Relieves liver and gall bladder pain that may occur after excessive ingestion of fatty foods, alcohol, coffee and chocolate. Should be taken by people exposed to aromatic hydrocarbons, solvents, paints, thinners, etc. Use when there are elevated liver enzymes (SGOT, SGPT), difficulty digesting fats, or during hepatitis flare-ups. Also for mild frontal headaches after fatty meals, for mild constipation and simple jaundice. Finally, it lowers high bilirubin levels.

Ingredients: *Milk Thistle, Toadflax, Oregon Grape, Echinacea, Licorice, Greater Celandine, Fringetree, Culver's root, Blue Flag.*

Dose: *Take 15-25 drops or one softgel two or three times a day.*

Contraindications: *Not in pregnancy.*

Lobelia (*Lobelia inflata*, dried herb in the bladder seed stage). Specific for bronchial spasms as may occur in asthma. Helps decrease craving for nicotine when quitting smoking.

Dose: *Take 5-20 drops not more than three times a day. Do not exceed recommended dosage.*

Contraindications: *Not in pregnancy.*

Side effects: *May cause nausea and vomiting.*

Warning: *Excessive amount slows heartbeat and depresses respiration.*

Lomatium (*Lomatium dissectum*, dried root). Used for lung problems, pneumonia, flu and fevers. Lomatium shortens the duration of respiratory viral infections. Very helpful with chronic fatigue immuno-dysfunction syndrome (CFIDS), Epstein-Barr virus and cytomegalovirus infection.

Dose: *Take 15-30 drops up to four times a day.*
Contraindications: *Not in pregnancy.*
Side effects: *May cause skin rash.*
Warning: *If skin rash occurs, cease use.*

Lung Tonic™ (Mullein/Horehound Complex). Specific support for chronic obstructive pulmonary disease (COPD), including emphysema, chronic bronchitis and asthma. Useful for congestion, inflammation of bronchioles and lung tissue, spasms of bronchioles and excessive production of mucus. Helps protect against respiratory infection, soothes and calms coughs. Ideal formula for long-term management of lung problems.
Ingredients: *Mullein, Horehound, Elecampane, Grindelia, Echinacea, Pleurisy Root, Passionflower, Osha, Lobelia, Yerba Santa.*
Dose: *Take 20-30 drops or one softgel three times a day. Specific for long-term use.*

Lymphatonic™ (Echinacea/Red Root Complex). Excellent deep acting immune system cleaner. A must for recurring or lingering, hard to shake colds, flu, infections and frequent minor illnesses. Use for acute swelling of tonsils and/or lymph nodes. Specific for uterine, ovarian or breast cysts. Speeds up healing of cuts, boils, or other poorly healing abrasions. Useful to shorten healing time of poison ivy or poison oak infection as well as cat-scratch disease.
Ingredients: *Echinacea, Red Root, Ocotillo, Burdock, Licorice, Dandelion, Yellow Dock, Wild Indigo, Blue Flag, Stillingia.*
Dose: *For acute symptoms, take 15-25 drops or one softgel every hour. In chronic stage, take 25-40 drops or one softgel two to three times day. For cysts, take with Red Root, 20 drops of each three times a day.*
Contraindications: *Not in pregnancy*

Maitake (*Grifola frondosa*, dried fruiting body and mycelium). An internal organ tonic, it protects and enhances the functioning of internal organs, including the heart, liver, kidneys, nervous system, lungs and stomach. It is also a cancer preventative and useful in treating chronic fatigue immuno-dysfunction syndrome (CFIDS).
Dose: *Take 20-30 drop twice a day for at least 100 days.*

Marshmallow (*Althaea officinalis*, fresh root). For any inflammation of the digestive system, such as the mouth, stomach, intestines and colon. Also soothes sore throats.
Dose: Take 20-40 drops up to five times a day.
Warning: May cause delayed absorption of other drugs taken at the same time.

Meadowsweet (*Filipendula ulmaria*, dried pre-flowering herb). Aspirin substitute. For inflammation of muscles or joints, rheumatic, arthritic and gout. Offers relief in heartburn, hyperacidity, nausea, cystitis, nephritis, menstrual cramps, gastritis and peptic ulcers. Helps in reducing fevers.
Dose: Take 15-25 drops up to four times a day.

Menopautonic™ (Dong Quai/Vitex Complex). Decreases or stops menopausal symptoms such as hot flashes, sweating, nervousness, insomnia, urinary frequency and back pain. Lifts menopausal depression within a week.
Ingredients: Dong Quai, Vitex, Hawthorn flowers, Black Cohosh, False Unicorn, Motherwort, Licorice, Passionflower, Siberian Ginseng, Pipsissewa, Cultivated American Ginseng, Dulse.
Dose: Take 20-30 drops or one softgel early morning and before retiring.
Contraindications: Not in pregnancy.

Migra-Free® (Feverfew/Periwinkle Complex). Migra-Free® is effective in migraine headache attacks. A truly wonderful preventative formula. Taken every day, it prevents inflammation of blood vessels in the brain and stops migraine headaches before they begin, even those headache attacks resistant to conventional medicines.
Ingredients: Feverfew, Periwinkle, Ginkgo, Meadowsweet, White Willow, Stevia.
Dose: During an acute migraine attack, take 40 drops every hour until migraine subsides. As a preventative, take 40 drops once a day. Can be taken for an unlimited period of time.

Milk Thistle (*Silybum marianum*, dried seed). The premier liver herb! Useful for chronic hepatitis, for fatty livers of alcoholics or even for cirrhosis of the liver. Protects the liver from harmful substances such

....

as alcohol, fumes and drugs, and stimulates its regeneration. Protects individuals who may come in long-term contact with chemicals, metals or aromatic hydrocarbons, such as solvents.

Dose: *Take 10-25 drops up to three times a day.*

Montezuma's ReLeaf™ (Sweet Annie/Quassia Complex). Prevents and counters amoebic, giardial or other types of parasitic infections where infection produces intestinal gas, diarrhea and mild to severe abdominal cramps. A must when traveling in foreign countries. Use when there is pain in the lower right abdomen, dull twinges with constipation or diarrhea, and poor fat digestion and absorption.

Ingredients: *Sweet Annie, Quassia, Oregon Grape, Bistort, Ginger, Angelica, Bayberry.*

Dose: *Against infection, take 15-30 drops every two to three hours. As a preventative, take 10 drops ten minutes before each meal.*

Contraindications: *Not in pregnancy.*

Monthly ReLeaf™ (Chaste Tree/Dandelion Complex). Symptoms associated with congestive dysmenorrhea (cyclic pain associated with menses). Decreases or eliminates dull or aching pelvic pain, pelvic congestion, sore and swollen breasts, abdominal distention, general water retention, swollen ankles and fingers, headaches, nausea, vomiting, constipation or diarrhea, fatigue, irritability, nervousness.

Ingredients: *Chaste Tree, Dandelion, Dong Quai, Motherwort, Horse Chestnut, Cramp Bark, Ginger.*

Dose: *Take 40-100 drops, or one-half to one teaspoon of the extract in warm water, every three or four hours beginning one or two days prior to menstruation until symptoms subside. If the congestion occurs every month, take one-half teaspoon three times a day up to one week before menstruation.*

Contraindications: *Not in pregnancy.*

Motherwort *(Leonurus cardiaca,* fresh flowering herb). Reduces water retention and menstrual cramps. Decreases the amount, length and severity of hot flashes and menopausal depression. Restores elasticity and secretion of post-menopausal vaginal walls. Also excellent for calming rapid heart beat, palpitation and hypertension from thyroid stress.

Dose: *Take 20-50 drops up to four times a day.*

Contraindications: *Not in pregnancy.*

Mouth Tonic™ (Myrrh/Goldenseal Complex). Used primarily as an external treatment for mouth and gum sores, bleeding gums, fever blisters, herpes sores and mouth ulcers (aphtous stomatitis), sores from dentures, enlarged and spongy tonsils and receding gums due to degeneration. Wonderful for pyorrhea and periodontal disease. May also be taken internally for colds and flu.

Ingredients: Echinacea, Myrrh, Goldenseal, Propolis, Yerba Mansa, Bloodroot.

Dose: Apply with cotton swab twice a day. Do not rinse. If stinging or irritation occurs, dilute with a little water. Internally: 20-30 drops every two to three hours.

M-Roid ReLeaf™ (Butcher's Broom/Collinsonia Complex). Useful for hemorrhoids, varicocele, prostatitis, urethritis, bladder irritation and acute bowel disorders, especially when there is a sense of constriction, pain and irritation in the pelvic area. This formula increases blood supply system drainage from the intestines, prostate and pelvic areas and relieves liver congestion (portal circulation congestion).

Ingredients: Butcher's Broom, Collinsonia, Horse Chestnut, Ocotillo, Red Root, Milk Thistle, Yellow Dock, Bogbean, Yarrow, Licorice, Stevia.

Dose: Take 20-30 drops twice a day for three weeks. Stop for one week. Repeat.

Contraindications: Not in pregnancy.

Mullein (*Verbascum thapsus*, fresh top leaf). Specific for coughs, especially in older asthmatic patients. Very useful for sub-acute or chronic bronchitis, emphysema or chronic obstructive pulmonary disease which worsens with nervousness.

Dose: Take 25-40 drops every three hours.

Mullein/Garlic Ear Drops FOR EXTERNAL USE ONLY. Specific to prevent or reduce middle ear infection (Otitis media). Acts as a gentle bacteriostatic, helps to reduce pain and assists in establishing the proper acidity/alkalinity ratio of the ear area.

Ingredients: Mullein flower, Garlic (fresh cloves and oil), in a base of Olive oil and Vitamin E.

Dose and usage directions: Warm the oil to body temperature, put 1-4 drops in each ear, insert sterile cotton in each ear to prevent dripping. Repeat every six to eight hours.

Contraindications: Not in perforated eardrums.
Warning: FOR EXTERNAL USE ONLY. Do not use in ears with perforated eardrums.

Mushrooms Seven Source™ (Reishi/Shiitake Complex). The ultimate medicinal mushroom formulation for those seeking a tonic containing only mushrooms. Similar to Deep Health™/Deep Chi Builder™ but with fewer adaptogenic properties. Deep immune system toner. Supports and strengthens all internal organs; lung, heart, liver, kidneys, stomach, pancreas, spleen, bladder, reproductive organs and intestines. Possesses strong anti-cancer and anti-tumor properties. Is used as a cancer preventative or during orthodox cancer therapy. Counteracts the negative effects of surgery, chemotherapy and radiation therapy. Stabilizes blood sugar problems. Helpful with nervousness, anxiety, sleeplessness, dizziness, chronic hepatitis, allergies, heart disease, high blood pressure, stomach and intestinal ulcers, as well as in chronic respiratory problems such as asthma, emphysema and bronchitis.

Ingredients: Reishi, Shiitake, Maitake, Oyster, Agaricus, Snow fungus, Cordyceps.
Dose: Take 20 to 30 drops twice a day for a minimum of one month. Best results are achieved by taking for 100 days or more.

Myrrh *(Commiphora myrrha,* gum exudate). For painful ulceration of the gums or mouth as in herpes or gingivitis, pharyngitis, sinusitis, laryngitis and indigestion. Taken in combination with Echinacea, Myrrh helps to elevate low white blood cell levels.
Dose: Take 10-20 drops four times a day.
Contraindications: Not in pregnancy. Not in overt kidney disease or excessive uterine bleeding.
Side effects: Large amounts may cause diarrhea and irritation of the kidneys.

Nervine Tonic™ (Passionflower/Valerian Complex). An excellent all-purpose daily sedative. Useful for soothing muscle twitches, nervousness, anxiety, nervous-type asthma, muscle pain or tightness from stress or overexertion, intestinal cramps. Useful while breaking the cycle of drug addiction. Helps to take the edge off pain. It decreases irritability of the nervous system and gently stimulates its repair.

Ingredients: *Passionflower, Valerian, Oat seed, Black Cohosh, Skullcap, Betony.*

Dose: *Take 15-50 drops or one softgel every three or four hour.*

Contraindications: *Not in pregnancy.*

Nettle, Stinging (*Urtica dioica*, fresh herb). Specific for hay fever and allergic rhinitis. Also for vaginitis, rheumatoid arthritis, stomatitis, eczema, diarrhea, hemorrhoids, asthma and gout. Tones up the mucous membranes especially where excessive mucus and inflammation are present. An alkalizing diuretic.

Dose: *For acute hay fever, 20 drops every half to one hour until relief is experienced, then take 20 drops four times a day. In other cases, 15-20 drops three times a day.*

Oat seed (*Avena sativa*, fresh seed in the milky stage). One of the best nervous system tonics available. Excellent for recuperating from a stressful experience or after an emotional breakdown. Helps in the withdrawal of nicotine, cocaine or opiates.

Dose: *Take 25 drops three times a day. Take for at least one month or more to achieve best results.*

Olive leaf (*Olea europaea*, dried leaf). Helpful in the beginning of bacterial, viral and fungal infections. Use for colds and flu, upper respiratory infection, ear infection, sinusitis. Recent studies have shown Olive leaf to be effective in herpes outbreaks reducing both the severity as well as healing time. Initial results suggest that it may be as effective as the drug acyclovir.

Dose: *Take 20-40 drops three to five times a day.*

Osha (*Ligusticum porteri*, dried root). A great herb at the beginning of a cold or flu. For early stages of: sore throat, chest cold with painful breathing, thick stringy mucus, or dry asthma. Stimulates the immune system and prevents secondary infections. Prevents recurrent middle ear infection in children; loosens and expels mucus.

Dose: *Take 20-40 drops three to four times a day.*

Contraindications: *Not in pregnancy.*

Osha Root Complex Syrup (Osha/Wild Cherry Complex). Stops or calms cough. Decreases lung congestion, promotes expectoration, and reduces inflammation of throat and bronchioles. Soothes and slightly anesthetizes the throat.

Ingredients: *Osha, Wild Cherry bark, White Pine, Balm of Gilead, Spikenard, and Bloodroot in a glycerin/gum arabic syrup base.*

Dose: *Take 1/2 to 1 teaspoon every three to four hours. Children, two to five years old, take 1/4 to 1/2 teaspoon every three to four hours.*

Contraindications: *Not during the first three months of pregnancy.*

Para-Free™ (Black Walnut/Wormwood Complex). This formula is designed to eliminate parasites such as giardia, entamoeba and other protozoal bugs. It inhibits pinworms and other types of parasites and tones up the digestive system.

Ingredients: *Fresh "green" Black Walnut, Wormwood, Quassia, Cloves, Male Fern.*

Dose: *Take 40 drops twice a day before meals.*

Contraindications: *Not in pregnancy or while breast-feeding.*

Passionflower (*Passiflora incarnata*, fresh flowering herb). For the "chattering" brain which prevents sleep. Calms the mind in headstrong individuals. Good for menopausal nervousness and anxiety, for persistent hiccough, and for frequent asthma attacks in children.

Dose: *For adults, 20-40 drops up to four times a day. For children five years and older, 10 drops up to four times a day.*

Passion Potion™ (Oats/Damiana Complex). Taken over time, an excellent sexual tonic for both men and women as it builds energy reserves. Stimulates a feeling of "well being." Specific for exhaustion, mild depression, chronic anxiety states, and/or during convalescence or any state of debility. Taken over time, increases stamina and decreases outbreaks of herpes and shingles. As a prelude to making love, it relaxes the mind and opens the heart.

Ingredients: *Oat seed, Damiana, Passionflower, Hawthorn flower, leaf and berry, Cultivated American Ginseng, Licorice, Stinging Nettle, Stevia, Parsley root.*

Dose: *Take 20-40 drops twice a day. Take for at least one month or more to achieve best results.*

Pau D'Arco (*Tabebuia impetiginosa*, Argentinian dried inner bark). **Internally:** Take for systemic candida infections, and fungal infections of the mouth (thrush). **Externally**: Use for fungal infection in feet, babies' bottoms or women's vaginas.
Dose: **Internally:** *Take 15-25 drops up to four times a day.* **Externally:** *Dilute with a little water and apply.*
Warning: For babies less than six months old, use EXTERNALLY only.

Pennyroyal (*Hedeoma pulegioides*, fresh pre-flowering herb). Specific for late, painful, spotty menstruation accompanied by sore breasts, bloating, and other PMS symptoms. Helps to induce delayed menstruation. Helps to break dry fever, calm coughs and stimulate mucus expectoration.
Dose: Take 20-40 drops in water three to four times a day. To stimulate sweating, take in hot water.
Contraindications: Not in pregnancy.

Peppermint (*Mentha piperita*, fresh pre-flowering herb). Stops nausea or vomiting. Stimulates the production and release of bile; prevents intestinal fermentation; stops gas formation. Stops stomach and intestinal cramping.
Dose: Take 10-20 drops after meals.

Phytocillin™ (Usnea/Hops Complex). Use for mouth, gum, stomach or intestinal infections. Respiratory infections including sinus, throat, lungs, bronchioles, respond rapidly to its use. Can be used internally for either gram positive or gram-negative bacterial infections as well as viral and fungal infections. Use externally for Staph, Strep or fungal infection, athlete's foot, ringworm or as a douche in Trichomonas infection. Also used externally for abrasions, skin ulcers, boils, pressure ulcers (i.e., bed sores), impetigo, skin infections or burns.
Ingredients: Usnea, Yerba Mansa, Propolis, Oregon Grape, Hops.
Dose: Take 30 to 90 drops or one to two softgels every two or three hours until the infection is no longer noticeable. Continue for 3 more days three times a day to ensure that the infection is completely gone. External use: Dilute and apply. For douching, one teaspoon of extract per pint of boiled water, cool and douche.
Contraindications: Not in pregnancy.

....

Warning: *If infection persists longer than three days or a fever is present, seek the advice of a primary care practitioner.*

Pipsissewa (*Chimaphila umbellata*, fresh herb). For bladder, kidney or urethra irritation or infection, especially after overindulging in alkaline foods, fruits and vegetables. Also for prostate irritation when dull pain occurs upon first urination in morning.
Dose: *Take 10-25 drops up to four times a day.*

Pleurisy Root (*Asclepias tuberosa*, dried root). As its name implies, useful in pleurisy, pneumonia, bronchitis or chest colds with dry respiratory membranes and skin. For dry skin problems, such as eczema or psoriasis.
Dose: *Take 15-30 drops three to four times a day.*
Contraindications: *Not in pregnancy.*
Side effects: *May cause nausea and vomiting.*

PMS ReLeaf™ (Vitex/Dandelion Complex). Stabilizes the emotional and physical components of PMS. Eliminates excess fluids; supports the liver; prevents build up of prostaglandins; stimulates fluid drainage from congested tissues (breasts and pelvic area). Reduces PMS symptoms such as water retention, swollen and tender breasts, lower backache, cramping, fatigue, irritability, insomnia, depression, difficulty in concentrating, panic attacks, anxiety, mood swings, crying, physical and emotional tension, low blood sugar, low sex drive, headaches and migraines.
Ingredients: *Vitex, Dandelion, Fringetree, Stinging Nettle, Red Root, Pulsatilla, Cramp Bark, Cleavers, Ginger, Stevia.*
Dose: *For acute symptoms, take 30 drops every three to four hours as needed. For chronic conditions or extreme PMS symptoms, take 30 drops three times a day beginning up to two weeks prior to menstruation. Also consider taking Cycle 1 Estrotonic™ and Cycle 2 Progestonic™. For painful cramping, also consider taking Cramp ReLeaf™ or Herbaprofen™.*
Contraindications: *Not in pregnancy.*

Propolis (Dry gum from beehives). For mouth, gum and intestinal infections; foul smelling diarrhea from intestinal infections. For skin abrasions, especially in moist areas such as feet, hands and face.

Dose: Internally: *Take 15-30 drops up to four times a day.* **Externally:** *Dilute and apply.*

Warning: *Should not be used internally by those with known reactions to bees or bee products, such as bee pollen or honey.*

Prostatonic™ (Saw Palmetto/Damiana Complex). Offers relief for benign enlargement of the prostate when enlargement has caused varying degrees of urinary problems such as frequent and urgent urination, difficulty in urinating or sensation of incomplete emptying of the bladder and dribbling. Helps reduce inflammation of these tissues and increases uptake of circulating male hormones. Also soothes genital pain caused by excessive sexual activity.

Ingredients: *Saw Palmetto, Yarrow, Dong Quai, Cultivated American Ginseng, Cleavers, Pipsissewa, Yerba Mansa, Sarsaparilla, Damiana, Kava, Nettle root.*

Dose: *Take 20-30 drops or one softgel two to three times a day for an unlimited period of time. Takes up to six weeks for effects to be noticeable.*

Red Clover (*Trifolium pratense*, fresh flower). High in minerals. Good as a maintenance liquid during infections, hepatitis or mononucleosis. Helps increase lactation in nursing mothers. Also helpful for psoriasis and eczema.

Dose: *Take 15-30 drops up to four times a day. Dosage for children: 10 drops up to four times a day.*

Contraindications: *Not in pregnancy.*

Red Raspberry (*Rubus idaeus,* fresh leaf). Used in pregnancy to prevent spotting during the first trimester and to increase overall muscle tone of the uterine walls. Also for excessive menstrual bleeding and mild diarrhea. Use diluted as a rinse for mouth ulcers and bleeding gums.

Dose: Internally: *Take 15-30 drops up to three times a day.* **Externally:** *Use diluted as a wash.*

Red Root (*Ceanothus americanus*, dried root and root bark). For acute tonsillitis or sore throat; inflamed spleen and/or inflamed lymphatic nodes, and fluid cysts in breasts, ovaries, uterus or testes.

Dose: *Take 20-40 drops up to four times a day. For cysts, take with Lymphatonic™, 20 drops of each three times a day.*

Reishi (*Ganoderma lucidum*, dried fruiting body and mycelium). Protects and enhances the functioning of internal organs, including the heart, liver, kidneys, nervous system, lungs and stomach. Long-term immune and nervous system tonic, assists in decreasing allergic reactions, cardiotonic and is showing excellent promise in cancer prevention and treatment research.

Dose: *Take 20-30 drop twice a day for at least 100 days.*

Remember Now™ (Ginkgo/Gotu Kola Complex). Specific for memory disorders, poor concentration and symptoms of primary cerebral arteriosclerosis, such as poor memory, irritability, restlessness, speech and motor (movement) disorders, vertigo, headaches and lack of attention. Has a positive effect on tinnitis, dizziness and hearing defects, especially when these occur in old age as a result of poor blood circulation. Also useful after strokes.

Ingredients: *Ginkgo, Periwinkle, Gotu Kola, Peppermint, Oat seed, St. John's Wort, Siberian Ginseng, Rosemary, Prickly Ash bark.*

Dose: *Take 20-30 drops or one softgel twice a day for an unlimited period of time. Takes up to six weeks for effects to be noticeable.*

Respiratonic™ (Osha/Pleurisy Root Complex). Relieves chest colds, lung congestion, acute bronchitis and pleurisy. All-purpose expectorant that loosens mucus, dilates the bronchioles and stimulates general resistance. Decreases excessive heat in the lungs, eases pain of coughing and liquefies mucus.

Ingredients: *Echinacea, Osha, Licorice, Yerba Mansa, Yerba Santa, Pleurisy Root, Grindelia, Ginger.*

Dose: *Take 10-25 drops or one softgel every two to three hours.*

Contraindications: *Not in pregnancy.*

Sarsaparilla (*Smilax spp.*, dried root). Useful in simple prostate enlargement. Increases elimination of urea and uric acid. Helpful in gout, herpes, many types of skin problems, rheumatism and sores. For moderate deficiencies of adrenal or gonad hormonal production.

Dose: *Take 15-20 drops three times a day.*

Saw Palmetto (*Serenoa repens*, dried berry). Specific for simple prostate enlargement. For difficulty urinating, especially with benign prostatic hypertrophy and dribbling of urine. Useful when reproductive glands are tender from excessive sexual activity.
Dose: *Take 20-30 drops up to four times a day for an unlimited period of time. It may take up to six weeks for effects to kick in.*

Schisandra (*Schisandra chinensis* [Wu wei zi], dried berry). Increases overall resistance. Helps fight stress, fatigue, tiredness, exhaustion and depression. Helps in allergic skin disorders. Considered nearly as good a general tonic as Ginseng.
Dose: *Take 15-25 drops twice a day for at least 100 days to achieve best results.*

Shepherd's Purse (*Capsella bursa-pastoris*, fresh herb). For excessive uterine bleeding or bleeding hemorrhoids. Specific for acute attacks of gout or any other conditions in which blood uric acid is elevated.
Dose: *Take 15-30 drops three times a day. For acute gout attack, take 30 drops every two hours for a day or two.*
Contraindications: *Not in pregnancy.*
Side effects: *Large doses of extract may cause heart palpitations.*
Warning: *If prolonged, significant or unusual bleeding occurs, seek medical attention. Individuals with a history of kidney stones should use cautiously.*

Shiitake (*Lentinus edodes*, dried fruiting body and mycelium). Supports and protects the immune system. Protects the heart by lowering elevated blood pressure and reducing very low-density lipoproteins (VLDL) and low-density lipoprotein (LDL) cholesterol. It has been shown to improve liver function, protect the liver from injury and help produce antibodies against hepatitis B. It is also a cancer preventative and useful in treating chronic fatigue immuno-dysfunction syndrome (CFIDS).
Dose: *Take 20-30 drop twice a day for at least 100 days.*

Singer's Saving Grace® (Collinsonia/Jack-in-the-pulpit Complex). Ideal for sore throats, laryngitis,

....

pharyngitis, hoarseness, cough, expectoration of thick mucus and a feeling of dryness in the throat. A blessing for singers, preachers, teachers or anybody with a sore throat from singing, screaming, cheering, shouting or talking loudly for a long period of time. Also for sore throats at the beginning of a cold or as an aftermath of a lung infection.

Ingredients: Yerba Mansa, Collinsonia, Licorice, Jack-in-the-pulpit, Propolis, Echinacea, Ginger and Osha (in Extra Strength Original only). Also available in Honey Lemon, Cool Mint and Cinnamon.

Dose: Spray two or three times directly into the mouth every one to four hours.

Skullcap (*Scutellaria lateriflora*, fresh flowering herb). For inability to sleep, edgy feelings, restlessness, phantom pains after amputation, muscle twitching, neuralgia, pain from shingles, and sciatica.

Dose: Take 20-40 drops up to four times a day.

Slippery Elm (*Ulmus rubra*, dried inner bark). Useful for gastritis, enteritis, colitis, mouth and throat inflammation, duodenal ulcers, and diarrhea.

Dose: Take 10-30 drops up to five times a day.

Smoke Free Drops™ (Lobelia/Oat Seeds Complex). Ideal herbal combination formula for those wishing to stop smoking. Decreases withdrawal symptoms, calms the nervous system, dilates the bronchioles and loosens mucus. It is not habit forming and greatly assists the determined person who wishes to stop smoking.

Ingredients: Lobelia, Oat seed, Licorice, Osha, Passionflower, Pleurisy Root, Grindelia, Mullein leaf, Ginger.

Dose: Take 20-30 drops or one softgel every two to three hours.

Contraindications: Not in pregnancy.

St. John's Wort (*Hypericum perforatum*, fresh and dry flower in the bud stage). Effective for depression, anxiety, agitation, insomnia, loss of interest, and excessive sleeping. Used to treat retro-viral infections such as HIV and AIDS (this last indication is still under investigation).

Dose: Take 15-40 drops three times a day. Must be taken for at least three months to impact depression.

Contraindications: Not for use with antidepressants.
Side effects: *May cause increased photosensitivity (which may lead to skin rash) in fair-skinned individuals.*
Warning: *May potentiate the effects of antidepressants. Although photosensitivity in human beings is rare, fair-skinned individuals should avoid excessive exposure to UV irradiation (e.g. sunlight; tanning). Do not use while taking any prescription drugs without the advice of your primary care practitioner.*

Stomach Tonic™ (Chamomile/Catnip Complex).

Offers immediate relief for bloating, gas cramps, pain after eating, stomach acidity, and helps to soothe pain of stomach ulcers. Sweetens the breath and dispels nausea and vomiting. For ulcerated stomach, take Stomach Tonic™ to ease pain and symptoms between meals and during the night. Use Digestonic™ before meals to tone and regulate the flow of stomach digestive juices.
Ingredients: *Chamomile, Catnip, Fennel, Lavender, Star Anise, Cardamom, Gentian, Angelica, Prickly Ash berry.*
Dose: *For adults, take 5-15 drops in a little water three times a day, after meals or before bedtime. For babies, give 1-2 drops, diluted in a liquid, up to three times a day, after meals or before bedtime.*
Contraindications: *Not in pregnancy.*
Note: *Safe for babies two months and older.*

Turmeric (Curcuma longa, dried rhizome). For

inflammation of muscles and synovial membranes of joints in osteoarthritis, rheumatoid arthritis, myositis and fibromyositis. It also protects the liver against toxic substances. Useful for gall bladder stones, and inflammation of the gall bladder and liver.
Dose: *Take 10-30 drops three times a day.*
Contraindications: *Not in pregnancy. Not for use in bile duct obstruction, stomach/duodenal ulcers or hyperacidity.*

Usnea (Usnea barbata, dried lichen). Specific for

pneumonia, pleurisy, bronchitis, sinusitis, cystitis, urethritis, sore and/or Strep throat. Used externally for Staph, Strep or fungal infection, impetigo, athlete's foot, ringworm or as a douche in Trichomonas infection.

....

Dose: Internally: *Take 20-40 drops three to five times a day.* **Externally:** *Use straight or diluted as a wash.*

Uva Ursi (*Arctostaphylos uva-ursi*, dried leaf). For acute cystitis and urethritis accompanied with sharp stabbing-like pain when urinating; kidney or bladder ulceration. For cystitis in paraplegics.
Dose: *Take 20-30 drops four to five times a day for up to one week to achieve best results.*
Contraindications: *Not in pregnancy. Not in individuals with a history of kidney disorders, irritated digestive conditions, and with acidic urine or in conjunction with remedies which produce acidic urine.*
Side effects: *May cause stomach irritation.*
Warning: *Not for prolonged use without consulting a primary care practitioner.*

Valerian (*Valeriana officinalis*, fresh Autumn-harvested root). For nervousness, anxiety, and stress-related hypertension. Use for insomnia, emotional depression, poor sleep from pain or trauma, and gastro-intestinal or uterine cramps, especially in the weakened person.
Dose: *Take 20-80 drops as needed.*

Vein Tonic™ (Horse Chestnut/Witch Hazel Complex). Specific for varicose veins, lymphedema, vascular spasms, chronic circulatory weakness and feeling of heaviness in the legs. Vein Tonic™ helps prevent cerebrovascular disease and thrombophlebitis. Relieves edema, reduces blood vessel permeability, increases venous and capillary tone and lessens inflammation of blood vessels. Relieves painful cramps in the legs at night and is recommended as a natural substitute for quinine medication.
Ingredients: *Horse Chestnut, Witch Hazel, Butcher's Broom, Rue, Sweet Clover, Calendula, Milk Thistle, Ocotillo, Oregon Grape, Stevia.*
Dose: *Take 25-35 drops twice a day for three weeks. Stop for one week. Repeat.*
Contraindications: *Not in pregnancy.*

Vitex (*Vitex agnus-castus* [Chaste Tree], dried berry). For premenstrual syndrome (PMS) caused by excess estrogen or low level of progesterone, menopausal change, and endometriosis. Also for acne and premenstrual herpes on the lips. Stimulates milk production in nursing mothers.

Dose: *Take 15-30 drops as needed. Best results are achieved if taken for a minimum of three to six months.*

Contraindications: *Not in pregnancy. Not while taking oral contraceptives.*

Warning: *May counteract the effectiveness of birth control pills.*

Wild Cherry (*Prunus serotina*, dried bark). Useful for irritating or chronic cough with excessive expectoration, bronchitis, or whooping cough. Also useful when recuperating from lung or digestive problems, pleurisy or pneumonia.

Dose: *Take 20-60 drops up to four times a day.*

Warning: *Not for long term use. Do not exceed recommended dose.*

Wild Yam (*Dioscorea villosa*, fresh root). Helps stop cramps or spasms of "hollow organs," such as intestines, gall bladder, uterus, bladder and ureters. Relieves inflammation in acute rheumatoid arthritis, and diverticulosis. Excellent for morning sickness. Helps ease stomach or intestinal irritability after operations.

Dose: *Take 20-40 drops four to five times a day.*

Side effects: *Large doses of the extract may cause vomiting.*

Yarrow (*Achillea millefolium*, fresh flowering herb). Taken in hot water, causes sweating and eases fever, symptoms of common colds, and amenorrhea (lack of menstruation). Taken in cold water, eases passive bleeding of the uterus, bladder or lungs; relieves gastric cramps, stomach gas, uterine spasms.

Dose: *Take 15-30 drops every four hours.*

Contraindications: *Not in pregnancy.*

Yeast ReLeaf™ (Pau D'Arco/Black Walnut Complex). For intestinal or systemic candida infection with resulting irregularities: diarrhea or constipation, bloating, low or fluctuating energy levels, vaginitis, menstrual difficulties, and/or allergic reactions to foods. Also used for thrush or mouth fungal infection, sinus infection, and certain types of eczema aggravated by candida. Useful on athlete's foot.

Ingredients: *Pau D'Arco, Quassia, Licorice, Echinacea, Myrrh, Yerba Mansa, Black Walnut, Thuja, Astragalus, Garlic.*
Dose: Internally: *Take 10-25 drops three to four times a day.* **Externally:** *Use straight, or diluted as a wash.*
Contraindications: *Not in pregnancy.*

Yellow Dock (*Rumex crispus*, dried root). For skin eruptions, acne, eczema, urticaria, psoriasis, accompanied by constipation, jaundice from liver congestion, bad breath and indigestion.
Dose: *Take 20-40 drops twice a day.*
Warning: *Use cautiously when a history of kidney stones is present.*

Yerba Mansa (*Anemopsis spp.*, dried root). Excellent substitute for Goldenseal. For slow healing conditions such as mouth, gum and throat sores, stomach and duodenal ulcers, colitis, pleurisy and bladder inflammation. Use externally for skin ulcers and boils. Use as a sitz bath for Bartholin gland cysts, perianal fissures and hemorrhoids.
Dose: Internally: *Take 20-40 drops up to four times a day.* **Externally:** *Dilute and apply.* **Sitz bath:** *Dilute one teaspoon per one quart of water.*

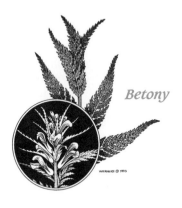

Betony

Health Condition Index

This index cross-references recommended herbs for health conditions listed in alphabetical order from A (Abdominal Pain) to Y (Yeast Infection). For detailed explanations of each recommended single herbal extract or formula, consult the **Herbal Directory** (Chapter 7).

   Please note: The herbs recommended for each health condition listed here are the herbs that are most appropriate and useful for that specific condition. For instance, when you read the **Herbal Directory** (Chapter 7), you will see that several herbs, such as Acnetonic™, Barberry, Chickweed, Dandelion, Echinacea, Gotu Kola, Vitex and Yellow Dock, are indicated in the treatment of acne. All are appropriate but in the interest of helping you choose the most useful herbs, this index limits its recommendations for acne to Acnetonic™, Dandelion, Vitex and Yellow Dock.

   As you consult this index, you may also notice that there are specialized conditions such as "decubitis" listed here that have not appeared previously in this book. Cat's Claw, for instance, is recommended here for decubitis. But in the **Herbal Directory** (Chapter 7), decubitis is not included in the description of Cat's Claw. Cat's Claw is, nevertheless, helpful for that condition. Listing every possible condition under every herb would have made the **Herbal Directory** (Chapter 7) too lengthy. Therefore, mention of rare or specialized conditions and their recommended herbs is limited to this index. Continue to follow the directions for use of recommended herbs as noted in the **Herbal Directory** (Chapter 7).

Abdominal pain

Chamomile
Montezuma's ReLeaf™
Peppermint
Stomach Tonic™

Abrasions, skin

Calendula (externally)
Phytocillin™
Propolis

Abscess

Dermatonic™
Lymphatonic™
Phytocillin™
Red Root

Acne

Acnetonic™
Dandelion
Vitex (around lips)
Yellow Dock
(on face and shoulders)

Acquired immune deficiency syndrome (AIDS), as support

Astragalus
Deep Health™
Licorice

Adaptogen

Adrenotonic™
Deep Health™
Ginsengs (American
& Siberian)
Ginseng Seven Source™

Addiction

Adrenotonic™
Oat seed

Adrenal

Adrenotonic™
Ginsengs (American
& Siberian)
Licorice

Agitation

Chamomile
Kava Cool Complex™
Kidalin®

Nervine Tonic™

Aids related complex (ARC)

Astragalus
Deep Health™
Licorice

Alcoholism

Liver Tonic™
Milk Thistle

Alertness

Bionic Tonic™
Ginkgo
Remember Now™

Allergic rhinitis

Allertonic™
Ephedra (Ma Huang)
Nettle, Stinging (fresh)

Allergic skin disorders

Allertonic™
Nettle, Stinging (fresh)

Allergies, acute

Allertonic™
Ephedra (Ma Huang)
Eyebright
Nettle, Stinging (fresh)

Allergies, prevention of

Adrenotonic™
Allertonic™
Deep Health™

Altitude adjustment

Chlorophyll Concentrate™

Alzheimer's disease

Ginkgo
Remember Now™

Amenorrhea (lack of menstruation)

Cycle 1 Estrotonic™
Cycle 2 Progestonic™

Amenorrhea, from travelling or stress

Pennyroyal

Amoebic infection
Barberry
Montezuma's ReLeaf™

Anemia
Alfalfa
Chlorophyll Concentrate™

Angina
Cardiotonic™
Hawthorn

Antihistamine
Allertonic™
Licorice
Nettle, Stinging (fresh)

Anxiety
Kava
Kava Cool Complex™
Nervine Tonic™
Valerian

Appetite, poor
Barberry
Digestonic™

Arrhythmia, heart
Cardiotonic™
Hawthorn

Arthritis
Arnica (externally)
Arthrotonic™
Devil's Claw

Arthritis, acute pain from
Herbaprofen™
Meadowsweet

Asthma, acute
Congest Free™
Decongestonic™
Ephedra (Ma Huang)
Lobelia

Asthma, chronic
Adrenotonic™
Lung Tonic™
Nettle, Stinging (fresh)

Athlete's foot
Usnea (externally)
Yeast ReLeaf™ (externally)

Attention deficit disorder (ADD)
Catnip
Kidalin®

Attention deficit hyperactivity disorder (ADHD)
Catnip
Kidalin®

Autoimmune disorders
Adrenotonic™
Deep Health™
Essiac Tonic™

Back pain
Herbaprofen™
Valerian

Back pain, from menstruation
PMS ReLeaf™

Bacterial infection
Echinacea
Echinacea Triple Source™
Goldenseal/Echinacea
    Complex
Phytocillin™
Usnea

Bartholin gland cyst
Lymphatonic™
Red Root
Yerba Mansa (externally)

Bed sores
Calendula (externally)
Lymphatonic™
Phytocillin™
Propolis

Bed wetting
California Poppy
Horsetail

Bile secretion

Dandelion
Liver Tonic™

Bilirubin, high levels of

Liver Tonic™

Birth pains, after

Black Cohosh
Cramp ReLeaf™

Bites, bug

Echinacea
(externally & internally)
Echinacea Triple Source™
(externally & internally)
Ivy Itch ReLeaf™
(externally)

Bitter tonic

Barberry
Digestonic™

Bladder irritation or infection

Cran-Bladder ReLeaf™
Kidney Tonic™
Uva Ursi

Bleeding

Red Raspberry
Shepherd's Purse

Blepharitis

Eyebright
(externally, diluted)

Bloating

Peppermint
Stomach Tonic™
Yeast ReLeaf™

Blood builder

Chlorophyll Concentrate™
Yellow Dock

Blood cholesterol, high

Cholesterotonic™
Deep Health™
Ginseng, Siberian

Blood cleanser

Burdock
Dandelion
Dermatonic™
Liver Tonic™

Blood poisoning

Echinacea
Echinacea Triple Source™
Lymphatonic™
Phytocillin™

Blood pressure, high

HB Pressure Tonic™
Passionflower

Blood sugar, high

Blueberry

Blood sugar, low

Adrenotonic™
Ginseng, Siberian
Licorice

Blood triglycerides, high

Cholesterotonic™
Deep Health™
Ginseng, Siberian

Boils

Burdock
Dermatonic™
Lymphatonic™

Breasts, sore

PMS ReLeaf™
Vitex

Bronchioles

Lung Tonic™
Mullein
Osha
Respiratonic™

Bronchitis, acute

Goldenseal/Echinacea
Complex
Osha
Phytocillin™
Respiratonic™

Bronchitis, chronic
Lung Tonic™
Mullein

Broncho-spasms
Adrenotonic™
Lobelia
Lung Tonic™
Respiratonic™

Bruise
Arnica (externally)

Burns, skin
Calendula (externally)
Lymphatonic™

Bursitis
Arthrotonic™
Cat's Claw
Herbaprofen™

Calcium absorption
Alfalfa
Nettle, Stinging (fresh)

Cancer, prevention of
Deep Health™
Essiac Tonic™
Red Clover

Cancer, support during treatment
Deep Health™
Essiac Tonic™

Candidiasis (candida)
Black Walnut
Cat's Claw
Yeast ReLeaf™

Canker sores
Goldenseal
Mouth Tonic™

Car sickness
Ginger

Cat scratch disease
Lymphatonic™

Catarrh (mucus)
Goldenseal
Goldenseal/Echinacea
Complex
Osha

Cerebrovascular disease, prevention of
Deep Health™
Vein Tonic™

Chemical exposure
Chaparral
Echinacea
Liver Tonic™

Chest cold
Echinacea
Echinacea Triple
Source Plus™
Goldenseal/Echinacea
Complex
Lymphatonic™
Osha
Respiratonic™

Childbirth
Black Cohosh
Blue Cohosh

Cholesterol, elevated
Cholesterotonic™
Deep Health™
Ginseng, Siberian

Chronic fatigue immuno-dysfunction syndrome (CFIDS)
Adrenotonic™
Essiac Tonic™
Lomatium

Chronic obstructive pulmonary disease (COPD)
Lung Tonic™
Mullein
Osha

Circulation

Cayenne
Ginkgo
Vein Tonic™

Cirrhosis

Liver Tonic™
Milk Thistle

Colds, first day

Echinacea
Echinacea Triple
  Source Plus™
Elderberry

Colds, prevention of

Deep Health™
Echinacea
Echinacea/Astragalus
  Complex
Echinacea Triple
  Source Plus™

Colds, unshakable

Lymphatonic™
Red Root

Colic

Chamomile
Peppermint
Stomach Tonic™

Colitis

Cat's Claw
Chamomile
Peppermint
Stomach Tonic™

Common cold

Echinacea
Echinacea Triple Source™
Goldenseal/Echinacea
  Complex
Osha
Phytocillin™
Respiratonic™

Common Cold, prevention of

Deep Health™
Echinacea/Astragalus
  Complex

Concentration

Ginkgo
Remember Now™

Congestion

Allertonic™
Congest Free™
Decongestonic™
Ephedra (Ma Huang)
Respiratonic™

Congestive heart failure

Cardiotonic™
Hawthorn

Conjunctivitis

Allertonic™
Eyebright
  (externally, diluted)

Constipation

Barberry
Liver Tonic™
Yellow Dock

Contraction, to stimulate uterine

Black Cohosh
Blue Cohosh

Convalescence

Deep Health™
Ginseng

Coughs

Osha
Osha Root
  Complex Syrup
Respiratonic™
Singer's Saving Grace®

Cramps, intestinal

Herbaprofen™
Peppermint
Stomach Tonic™

Cramps, in legs at night

Vein Tonic™

Cramps, menstrual

Black Cohosh
Cramp ReLeaf™

Herbaprofen™
Monthly ReLeaf™
PMS ReLeaf™

Crohn's disease

Cat's Claw
Chamomile
Peppermint

Cuts, infected

Hops
Phytocillin™
Usnea

Cuts, slow healing

Deep Health™
Lymphatonic™
Propolis (externally)

Cystitis

Cran-Bladder ReLeaf™
Kidney Tonic™
Uva Ursi

Cysts, breast,
ovarian or uterine

Lymphatonic™
Red Root

Cytomegalovirus
infection

Astragalus
Deep Health™
Lomatium

Dandruff

Burdock
Dermatonic™

Debility

Adrenotonic™
Deep Health™
Passion Potion™

Decubitis (Bed Sores)

Cat's Claw
Chamomile
Lymphatonic™
  (internally)
Phytocillin™

Dentures, sores from

Goldenseal
Mouth Tonic™
Myrrh

Deodorizer, intestinal

Chlorophyll Concentrate™

Depression

Damiana
Deprezac™
Passion Potion™
St. John's Wort

Depression,
with anxiety

Kava Cool Complex™

Dermatitis

Dandelion
Dermatonic™
Lymphatonic™

Diabetes, adult onset

Blueberry
Ginkgo

Diarrhea

Bayberry
Montezuma's ReLeaf™
Para-Free™
Propolis
Yeast ReLeaf™

Digestion, poor

Barberry
Digestonic™

Diuretic

Chickweed
Dandelion
Kidney Tonic™

Diverticulitis

Cat's Claw
Digestonic™
Peppermint

Dizziness

Ginger
Ginkgo
Remember Now™

Drug therapy, support during
- Adrenotonic™
- Deep Health™

Duodenal ulcers
- Chamomile
- Stomach Tonic™

Dysentery
- Cat's Claw
- Montezuma's ReLeaf™
- Para-Free™

Dyspepsia
- Chamomile
- Peppermint
- Stomach Tonic™

Ears
- Ginkgo
- Mullein/Garlic Ear Drops
- Osha

Earache, from congestion
- Congest Free™
- Ephedra (Ma Huang)
- Goldenseal/Echinacea Complex

Ear infection
- Goldenseal/Echinacea Complex
- Mullein/Garlic Ear Drops
- Phytocillin™

Ear infection, recurrent
- Lymphatonic™
- Osha

Eczema
- Burdock
- Dandelion
- Dermatonic™
- Nettle, Stinging (fresh)

Emphysema
- Lung Tonic™
- Mullein

Endometriosis
- Cycle 2 Progestonic™
- Vitex

Endurance, lack of
- Adrenotonic™
- Astragalus
- Deep Health™

Energy
- Adrenotonic™
- Bionic Tonic™
- Deep Health™
- Ginsengs, all

Entamoeba
- Black Walnut
- Para-Free™

Enteritis
- Chamomile
- Peppermint
- Stomach Tonic™

Epstein-Barr virus
- Astragalus
- Deep Health™
- Echinacea/Astragalus Complex
- Lomatium

Estrogen deficiency
- Black Cohosh
- Cycle 1 Estrotonic™
- Dong Quai

Exhaustion
- Adrenotonic™
- Deep Health™
- Ginsengs, all
- Ginseng Seven Source™
- Oat seed

Expectorant
- Osha
- Osha Root Complex Syrup
- Respiratonic™

Extremities, cold
- Cayenne
- Ginger

Eye

Eyebright
(externally, diluted &
internally)

Eyes, mild infection

Eyebright
(externally, diluted &
internally)
Phytocillin™
(externally, diluted &
internally)

Fasting

Alfalfa
Burdock
Lymphatonic™

Fatigue

Adrenotonic™
Astragalus
Bionic Tonic™
Deep Health ™
Ginseng Seven Source™
Ginseng, Woodsgrown
American

Fatty liver

Liver Tonic™
Milk Thistle

**Fermentation,
intestinal**

Peppermint
Stomach Tonic™

Fertility, low female

Cycle 1 Estrotonic™
Cycle 2 Progestonic™
Dong Quai
Vitex

Fertility, low male

Prostatonic™
Saw Palmetto

Fever

Goldenseal/Echinacea
Complex
Herbaprofen™
Meadowsweet

**Fibroid cysts, breast,
uterus, ovarian**

Lymphatonic™
Red Root
Vitex

Fibromyalgia

Herbaprofen™
Turmeric

Fibrositis

Arthrotonic™
Devil's Claw
Herbaprofen™
Turmeric

Flatulence

Chamomile
Peppermint
Stomach Tonic™

Flu

Echinacea Triple
Source Plus™
Elderberry
Goldenseal/Echinacea
Complex
Osha

**Free radicals
scavenger**

Ginkgo
Remember Now™

Fungal infection

Black Walnut
Phytocillin™
Usnea
Yeast ReLeaf™

Gall bladder

Dandelion
Liver Tonic™
Turmeric

Gallstones, mild

Herbaprofen™
Liver Tonic™

Gas

Fennel
Peppermint
Stomach Tonic™

Gastric ulcers
Chamomile
Licorice
Stomach Tonic™

Gastritis/ gastroenteritis
Cat's Claw
Chamomile
Goldenseal
Stomach Tonic™

Giardial infection
Barberry
Montezuma's ReLeaf™
Para-Free™

Gingivitis
Mouth Tonic™
Myrrh
Propolis

Gout
Arthrotonic™
Cholesterotonic™
Devil's Claw
Shepherd's Purse

Gums
Mouth Tonic™
Myrrh
Propolis

Hay fever
Adrenotonic™
Allertonic™
Decongestonic™
Ephedra (Ma Huang)
Eyebright
Nettle, Stinging (fresh)

Hay fever, prevention
Adrenotonic™
Allertonic™
Deep Health™
Nettle, Stinging (fresh)

Head cold
Congest Free™
Decongestonic™
Goldenseal/Echinacea
  Complex

Headache, acute
Feverfew
Herbaprofen™
Meadowsweet
Migra-Free®

Headache, chronic
Feverfew
Liver Tonic™
Migra-Free®

Hearing disorders
Ginkgo
Remember Now™

Heartburn
Peppermint
Stomach Tonic™

Heart support
Cardiotonic™
Hawthorn
Motherwort

Heart tonic
Cardiotonic™
Deep Health™
Hawthorn
Reishi

Hemorrhoids
Cat's Claw
M-Roid ReLeaf™

Hepatitis
Deep Health™
Liver Tonic™
Milk Thistle

Herpes
Cat's Claw
Echinacea
Echinacea Triple Source™
Lymphatonic™
Mouth Tonic™
Vitex (on lips)

Hiccough
Passionflower
Stomach Tonic™

High altitude sickness
Chlorophyll Concentrate™
Schisandra

High blood pressure

HB Pressure Tonic™
Passionflower

High density lipo-proteins (HDL)

Cholesterotonic™

Hives

Allertonic™
Ivy Itch ReLeaf™
(externally)
Nettle, Stinging (fresh)

Hoarseness

Osha
Singer's Saving Grace®

Hormone, imbalance

Cycle 1 Estrotonic™
Cycle 2 Progestonic™
Dong Quai
Vitex

Hormone, shift

Black Cohosh
Cycle 1 Estrotonic™
Cycle 2 Progestonic™
Menopautonic™
Vitex

Hormone, shift with skin flare up

Acnetonic™
Cycle 1 Estrotonic™
Cycle 2 Progestonic™
Vitex

Hot flashes

Dong Quai
Menopautonic™
Motherwort

Human immuno-deficiency virus (HIV)

Deep Health™
Echinacea
Echinacea/Astragalus
Complex
Echinacea Triple Source™
St. John's Wort

Hyperactivity

Catnip
Chamomile
Kidalin®

Hyperactivity, in children

Catnip
Kidalin®

Hyperglycemia (high blood sugar)

Blueberry

Hypersecretion, of mucus

Allertonic™
Decongestonic™
Ephedra (Ma Huang)
Goldenseal

Hypertension

HB Pressure Tonic™
Passionflower

Hypochondria

Adrenotonic™
Deep Health™
Nervine Tonic™

Hypoglycemia

Adrenotonic™
Ginseng, Siberian
Licorice

Illness, recuperating from

Deep Health™
Ginsengs, all
Lymphatonic™

Immune system

Astragalus
Deep Health™
Echinacea
Echinacea/Astragalus
Complex
EchinaceaTriple Source™
Lymphatonic™

Impetigo

Echinacea Triple
  Source Plus™
Lymphatonic™
Phytocillin™
  (externally & internally)
Usnea
  (externally & internally)

Implantation, egg

Cycle 2 Progestonic™

Impotence

Prostatonic™
Saw Palmetto

Indigestion

Chamomile
Stomach Tonic™

Infants, colic

Chamomile
Stomach Tonic™

Infection

Echinacea
Echinacea Triple
  Source Plus™
Phytocillin™
Propolis
Usnea

Infection, recurring

Lymphatonic™
Red Root

Inflammation

Arthrotonic™
Devil's Claw
Herbaprofen™

Insect bites

Echinacea
  (externally & internally)
Echinacea Triple Source™
  (externally & internally)
Ivy Itch ReLeaf™
  (externally)
Lymphatonic™
  (internally)

Insomnia

California Poppy
Chamomile
Deep Sleep®
Kava Cool Complex™
Passionflower
Valerian

Intercourse, painful

Cycle 1 Estrotonic™
Cycle 2 Progestonic™
Menopautonic™

Intercourse, urinary infection after

Cran-Bladder ReLeaf™
Kidney Tonic™
Pipsissewa

Interferon, production of

Astragalus
Deep Health™
Echinacea
Echinacea/Astragalus
  Complex
Echinacea Triple Source™

Intestinal distress

Montezuma's ReLeaf™
Para-Free™
Peppermint

Intestines

Montezuma's ReLeaf™
Para-Free™
Peppermint

Irritable bowel syndrome

Deep Health™
Peppermint

Jaundice

Dandelion
Liver Tonic™

Jaw, tense

Kava
Kava Cool Complex™
Nervine Tonic™

Joints
  Arthrotonic™
  Devil's Claw
  Herbaprofen™
Kidney
  Dandelion
  Kidney Tonic™
Labor (to activate)
  Black Cohosh
  Blue Cohosh
Lactation
  Fennel
  Red Clover
  Vitex
Laryngitis
  Collinsonia
  Osha
  Singer's Saving Grace®
Leaky bowel syndrome
  Cat's Claw
  Para-Free™
  Yeast ReLeaf™
Leukorrhea
  Echinacea
  Echinacea Triple Source Plus™
  Pau D'Arco
  Yeast ReLeaf™
Lichen
  Black Walnut
  Phytocillin™
  Usnea
  Yeast ReLeaf™
Ligaments
  Echinacea
  Echinacea Triple Source™
Liver
  Barberry
  Dandelion
  Liver Tonic™
  Milk Thistle

Low density lipo-proteins (LDL)
  Cholesterotonic™
Lungs, congested
  Osha
  Respiratonic™
Lungs, weak
  Deep Health™
  Lung Tonic™
  Mullein
Lupus, support in
  Deep Health™
  Lymphatonic™
  Reishi
Lymph nodes, swollen
  Echinacea
  Echinacea Triple Source™
  Lymphatonic™
  Red Root
Lymphedema
  Lymphatonic™
  Red Root
Memory, to improve
  Ginkgo
  Gotu Kola
  Remember Now™
Menopause
  Black Cohosh
  Dong Quai
  Menopautonic™
  Motherwort
  Vitex
Menstrual cramps
  Black Cohosh
  Cramp ReLeaf™
  Monthly ReLeaf™
  Motherwort
  PMS ReLeaf™
Menstrual cycle, balancing
  Cycle 1 Estrotonic™
  Cycle 2 Progestonic™

Menstruation, delayed
- Damiana
- Pennyroyal

Menstruation, excessive bleeding during
- PMS ReLeaf™
- Red Raspberry
- Shepherd's Purse

Menstruation, general
- Cycle 1 Estrotonic™
- Cycle 2 Progestonic™
- Dong Quai
- Vitex

Metabolism, balance
- Adrenotonic™
- Deep Health™

Metal exposure
- Chaparral
- Liver Tonic™

Middle ear infection
- Echinacea/Astragalus Complex
- Goldenseal
- Goldenseal/Echinacea Complex
- Mullein/Garlic Ear Drops
- Osha
- Phytocillin™

Middle ear infection (recurring)
- Echinacea/Astragalus Complex
- Lymphatonic™
- Osha

Migraine headache
- Feverfew
- Migra-Free®
- PMS ReLeaf™

Milk production
- Fennel
- Red Clover
- Vitex

Miscarriage, prevention of
- Cramp ReLeaf™
- Wild Yam

Mononucleosis
- Liver Tonic™
- Milk Thistle
- Passion Potion™

Mood elevator
- Damiana
- Deprezac™
- Kava
- Kava Cool Complex™
- St. John's Wort

Morning sickness
- Cramp ReLeaf™
- Ginger
- Wild Yam

Motion sickness
- Ginger

Mouth
- Mouth Tonic™
- Myrrh
- Propolis

Mucous membranes
- Allertonic™
- Ephedra (Ma Huang)
- Goldenseal

Mucus, excess
- Goldenseal
- Goldenseal/Echinacea Complex
- Respiratonic™

Muscles
- Arnica (externally)
- Arthrotonic™
- Kava Cool Complex™
- Herbaprofen™

Myositis
- Arthrotonic™
- Herbaprofen™
- Turmeric

Nausea

Ginger
Stomach Tonic™

Nephritis

Kidney Tonic™
Marshmallow

Nervousness

Chamomile
Kava
Kava Cool Complex™
Nervine Tonic™
Oat seed
Valerian

Nervous system, exhaustion

Adrenotonic™
Deep Health™
Nervine Tonic™
Oat seed

Nervous system, hyperactivity

Kidalin®
Nervine Tonic™
Skullcap
Valerian

Neuralgia

Feverfew
Herbaprofen™
Nervine Tonic™
Valerian

Neuritis

Herbaprofen™
Nervine Tonic™
Skullcap
St. John's Wort

Nicotine withdrawal

Licorice
Lobelia
Oat seed
Smoke Free Drops™

Opiate withdrawal

Adrenotonic™
Oat seed

Osteoporosis

Arthrotonic™
Horsetail

Otitis media, acute

Echinacea/Astragalus
    Complex
Goldenseal/Echinacea
    Complex
Lymphatonic™
Mullein/Garlic Ear Drops
Osha
Phytocillin™

Otitis media, preventative

Echinacea/Astragalus
    Complex
Lymphatonic™
Osha

Ovarian cyst

Lymphatonic™
Red Root
Vitex

Ovaries

Black Cohosh
Cycle 1 Estrotonic™
Cycle 2 Progestonic™
Dong Quai

Over-exertion, muscle

Arnica (externally)
Herbaprofen™

Ovulation, enhancer

Cycle 1 Estrotonic™

Pain

Arthrotonic™
Black Cohosh
Herbaprofen™
Nervine Tonic™
Valerian

Palpitations

Cardiotonic™
Hawthorn
Motherwort

Pancreas
Blueberry
Licorice

Panic attack
Deprezac™
Kava
Kava Cool Complex™
St. John's Wort

Parasitic infection
Barberry
Montezuma's ReLeaf™
Para-Free™

Peptic ulcer
Cat's Claw
Chamomile
Stomach Tonic™

Perianal fissure
M-Roid ReLeaf™
Yerba Mansa (externally)

Periodontal disease
Goldenseal
Mouth Tonic™
Myrrh

Pharyngitis
Myrrh
Osha
Singer's Saving Grace®

Phlebitis
Arnica (externally)
Vein Tonic™

Pimples
Acnetonic™
Burdock
Dandelion
Dermatonic™
Lymphatonic™

Pinworms
Black Walnut
Para-Free™

Pleurisy
Osha
Phytocillin™

Pleurisy Root
Respiratonic™

Pneumonia
Lomatium
Osha
Phytocillin™
Respiratonic™

Poison ivy/oak
Echinacea Triple Source™
Ivy Itch ReLeaf™
Lymphatonic™

Post partum hemorrhage
Cramp ReLeaf™
Shepherd's Purse

Pregnancy, support
Red Raspberry

Pregnant, to get
Cycle 1 Estrotonic™
Cycle 2 Progestonic™
Dong Quai
Vitex

Premenstrual syndrome (PMS)
Dong Quai
Monthly ReLeaf™
PMS ReLeaf™
Vitex

PMS, water retention from
Chickweed
Dandelion
Kidney Tonic™
Monthly ReLeaf™
PMS ReLeaf™

Progesterone deficiency
Cycle 1 Estrotonic™
Cycle 2 Progestonic™
Vitex

Prostatitis
Prostatonic™
Saw Palmetto

Protozoal infection
Black Walnut
Para-Free™
Montezuma's ReLeaf™

Psoriasis
Burdock
Dandelion
Dermatonic™
Liver Tonic™

Psychoactive herbs
Deprezac™
Kava
Kava Cool Complex™
St. John's Wort

Pyorrhea
Goldenseal
Mouth Tonic™
Myrrh
Propolis

Red blood cells, low
Chlorophyll Concentrate™

Rejuvenation
Adrenotonic™
Deep Health™
Ginseng Seven Source™

Relaxation
Chamomile
Kava
Kava Cool Complex™
Nervine Tonic™

Respiratory system, support
Chlorophyll Concentrate™
Deep Health™
Lung Tonic™

Restlessness
Kava
Kava Cool Complex™
Kidalin®
Nervine Tonic™
Skullcap

Rheumatic condition
Arthrotonic™
Devil's Claw
Herbaprofen™

Rhinitis
Allertonic™
Congest Free™
Decongestonic™
Ephedra (Ma Huang)
Nettle, Stinging (fresh)

Ringworm
Black Walnut
Yeast ReLeaf™

Sciatica
Herbaprofen™
Nervine Tonic™
Skullcap
Valerian

Sea sickness
Ginger

Seasonal affective disorder (SAD)
Deprezac™
St. John's Wort

Sedative
California Poppy
Deep Sleep®
Nervine Tonic™
Valerian

Sexual energy, to decrease
Hops

Sexual tonic, for men
Damiana
Deep Health™
Passion Potion™
Saw Palmetto

Sexual tonic, for women
Damiana
Deep Health™
Dong Quai
Passion Potion™

Shingles

Herbaprofen™
Nervine Tonic™
Skullcap

Sinusitis

Congest Free™
Decongestonic™
Goldenseal
Nettle, Stinging (fresh)

Skin

Acnetonic™
Burdock
Dermatonic™

Skin, sores

Burdock
Dermatonic™
Lymphatonic™
Yellow Dock

Sleeping, excessive

Deep Health™
Deprezac™
St. John's Wort

Sleeping, problems

California Poppy
Chamomile
Deep Sleep®
Kava Cool Complex™
Passionflower
Valerian

Smoking, withdrawal

Adrenotonic™
Lobelia
Oat seed
Smoke Free Drops™

Solvent exposure

Chaparral
Liver Tonic™
Milk Thistle

Sore throat

Osha
Osha Root
Complex Syrup

Respiratonic™
Singer's Saving Grace®

Spasms, muscles

Feverfew
Herbaprofen™
Nervine Tonic™
Valerian

Spleen

Lymphatonic™
Red Root

Spotting in pregnancy, prevention of

Red Raspberry

Sprain

Arnica (externally)
Herbaprofen™

Staph infection

Goldenseal/Echinacea
  Complex
Phytocillin™
Usnea

Steroids, withdrawal or substitute

Adrenotonic™
Licorice
Sarsaparilla

Stimulant

Bionic Tonic™
Ginseng, Chinese Kirin Red

Sting, insects

Echinacea
  (externally & internally)
Echinacea Triple Source™
  (internally & externally)
Ivy Itch ReLeaf™
  (externally)

Stomach

Chamomile
Digestonic™
Peppermint
Stomach Tonic™

Stones, gall bladder
Liver Tonic™
Turmeric

Strain
Arnica (externally)
Herbaprofen™

Strep infection
Phytocillin™
Usnea

Stress
Adrenotonic™
Deep Health™
Ginsengs, all
Kava Cool Complex™
Nervine Tonic™
Passionflower
Valerian

Stroke
Cardiotonic™
Ginkgo
Hawthorn
Remember Now™

Stye
Echinacea
Echinacea Triple
Source Plus™
Eyebright
(externally, diluted)
Lymphatonic™

Surgery, recuperating from
Adrenotonic™
Deep Health™
Ginsengs, all

Swelling
Chamomile (externally)
Echinacea
Echinacea Triple Source™
Lymphatonic™

Synovial inflammation
Arthrotonic™
Devil's Claw
Herbaprofen™

Tachycardia
Cardiotonic™
Hawthorn
Motherwort

Tendonitis
Echinacea
Echinacea Triple Source™
Herbaprofen™

Tennis elbow
Echinacea
Echinacea Triple Source™
Herbaprofen™

Testosterone, high
Hops
Vitex

Testosterone, low
Prostatonic™
Saw Palmetto

Throat, sore
Osha
Osha Root
Complex Syrup
Respiratonic™
Singer's Saving Grace®

Throat, strep
Goldenseal/Echinacea
Complex
Phytocillin™
Usnea

Thrombophlebitis
Cardiotonic™
Vein Tonic™

Thrush
Black Walnut
Mouth Tonic™
Pau D'Arco
Phytocillin™
Yeast ReLeaf™

Thyroid gland
Gotu Kola

Tinnitis
Ginkgo
Remember Now™

Tiredness

Adrenotonic™
Deep Health™
Ginsengs, all
Schisandra

Tonic, general

Deep Health™
Ginsengs, all
Ginseng Seven Source™

Tonsillitis

Lymphatonic™
Phytocillin™
Red Root

Toothache

Echinacea
Herbaprofen™

Tranquilizer

Kava
Kava Cool Complex™
Nervine Tonic™
Valerian

Trichomoniasis

Black Walnut
Lymphatonic™
Yeast ReLeaf™

Triglycerides, high

Cholesterotonic™
Ginseng Seven Source™
Ginseng, Siberian
Ginseng, Woodsgrown
  American

Tumors

Deep Health™
Essiac Tonic™

Twitching, muscle

Nervine Tonic™
Skullcap

Ulceration

Chamomile
Goldenseal
Myrrh
Phytocillin™
Yerba Mansa

Ulcers, external and/or internal

Cat's Claw
Chamomile
Licorice
Yerba Mansa

Urethritis

Cran-Bladder ReLeaf™
Kidney Tonic™
Uva Ursi

Uric acid, to decrease

Arthrotonic™
Burdock
Devil's Claw
Shepherd's Purse

Urinary tract infection (UTI)

Cran-Bladder ReLeaf™
Kidney Tonic™
Uva Ursi

Urticaria

Allertonic™
Lymphatonic™
Nettle, Stinging (fresh)

Uterine contraction, weak

Black Cohosh
Blue Cohosh

Uterine cysts (fibroids)

Lymphatonic™
Red Root

Uterus

Black Cohosh
Cramp ReLeaf™
Cycle 1 Estrotonic™
Cycle 2 Progestonic™
Dong Quai

Vagina, dry

Black Cohosh
Cycle 1 Estrotonic™
Cycle 2 Progestonic™
Dong Quai
Menopautonic™
Vitex

Varicocele
  M-Roid ReLeaf™

Varicose veins
  Vein Tonic™

Vertigo
  Ginger
  Ginkgo
  Remember Now™

Viral infection
  Echinacea
  Echinacea Triple
    Source Plus™
  Elderberry
  Lomatium
  Osha
  Phytocillin™

Vitality, low
  Adrenotonic™
  Deep Health™
  Ginsengs, all
  Ginseng Seven Source™

Vomiting
  Ginger
  Peppermint
  Stomach Tonic™

Warts
  Black Walnut
  Phytocillin™
  Yeast ReLeaf™

Water retention
  Dandelion
  Kidney Tonic™
  PMS ReLeaf™

Weakness
  Adrenotonic™
  Astragalus
  Deep Health™

White blood cells, low
  Echinacea
  Echinacea Triple Source™
  Lymphatonic™
  Myrrh

Wound
  Echinacea
  Phytocillin™
  Usnea

Yeast infection
  Black Walnut
  Pau D'Arco
  Phytocillin™
  Yeast ReLeaf™

Lemon Balm

WERNEKE © 1993

Latin Name-

Common Name Index

Notes on the use of this index:

If you only know the Latin name of an herb, this index will help you find the common name so that you can look it up under its common name in the **Herbal Repertory** (Chapter 7).

Achillea millefolium	YARROW
Althaea officinalis	MARSHMALLOW
Anemopsis spp.	YERBA MANSA
Angelica sinensis	DONG QUAI
Arctium lappa	BURDOCK
Arctostaphylos uva-ursi	UVA URSI
Arnica spp.	ARNICA
Asclepias tuberosa	PLEURISY ROOT
Astragalus membranaceus	ASTRAGALUS
Avena sativa	OAT SEED
Berberis vulgaris	BARBERRY
Calendula officinalis	CALENDULA
Capsella bursa-pastoris	SHEPHERD'S PURSE
Capsicum annuum	CAYENNE
Caulophyllum thalictroides	BLUE COHOSH
Ceanothus americanus	RED ROOT
Centella asiatica	GOTU KOLA
Chimaphila umbellata	PIPSISSEWA
Cimicifuga racemosa	BLACK COHOSH
Collinsonia canadensis	COLLINSONIA
Commiphora myrrha	MYRRH
Crataegus spp.	HAWTHORN
Curcuma longa	TURMERIC
Dioscorea villosa	WILD YAM
Echinacea angustifolia	ECHINACEA
Eleutherococcus senticosus	SIBERIAN GINSENG
Ephedra sinica	EPHEDRA (MA HUANG)
Equisetum arvense	HORSETAIL
Eschscholzia californica	CALIFORNIA POPPY
Euphrasia officinalis	EYEBRIGHT
Filipendula ulmaria	MEADOWSWEET
Foeniculum vulgare	FENNEL
Ganoderma lucidum	REISHI
Gentiana lutea	GENTIAN
Ginkgo biloba	GINKGO

Ulmus rubra	SLIPPERY ELM
Uncaria tomentosa	CAT'S CLAW
Urtica dioica	NETTLE, STINGING
Usnea barbata	USNEA
Vaccinium spp.	BLUEBERRY
Valeriana officinalis	VALERIAN
Verbascum thapsus	MULLEIN
Viburnum opulus	CRAMP BARK
Vitex agnus-castus	VITEX (CHASTE TREE)
Withania somnifera	ASHWAGANDHA
Zingiber officinale	GINGER

The following two herbal extracts do not have Latin names:
CHLOROPHYLL & PROPOLIS

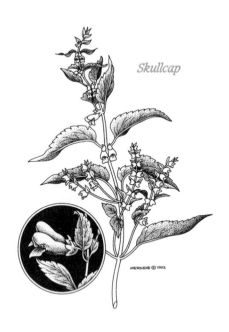

Skullcap

WERNEKE © 1993

Suggested Reading

For the lay person:

The following authors present useful and practical information and their books can be purchased at most natural product stores:

Daniel Gagnon and Amadea Morningstar

Breathe Free

This book was written because I wanted to share practical information on how to treat respiratory problems. My frustration with most existing herbal books is that they tell you which herbs to use, but not how much to take and why. Therefore, *Breathe Free* gives you specifics on which foods, supplements and herbs to take. It covers such problems as common colds and flu, hay fever, sore throats, earaches, asthma, pneumonia, bronchitis and emphysema, among other problems.

Christopher Hobbs

> *Echinacea, The Immune Herb*
> *Foundation of Health*
> *Ginkgo, Elixir of Youth*
> *Handbook for Herbal Healing*
> *Milk Thistle, The Liver Herb*
> *Natural Liver Therapy*
> *Medicinal Mushrooms*
> *Usnea, The Herbal Antibiotic*
> *Valerian, The Relaxing and Sleep Herb*
> *Vitex, The Women's Herb*

Christopher is a friend of mine. His books strike a good balance between imparting high-level scientific research and translating those research results into practical information for everyday use.

David Hoffmann

> *The New Holistic Herbal*
> *The Elder's Herbal*

Should you buy just one other herbal book for your family (in addition to *Liquid Herbal Drops in Everyday Use*), I would strongly suggest that it be David's *New Holistic Herbal.* Due to its comprehensive approach and well-organized chapters, I encourage my herbal medicine students to read this book.

Michael Moore

> *Medicinal Plants of the Desert and Canyon West*
> *Medicinal Plants of the Mountain West*
> *Medicinal Plants of the Pacific West*

Michael's great sense of humor turns what could be even the most potentially boring reading into an interesting experience. In his book *Medicinal Plants of the Pacific West*, for instance, his comparison of an herb called Western Skunk Cabbage to the carnivorous plant in the movie *Little Shop of Horrors* is quite a humorous review of this herb. Michael's incredible knowledge of physiology and profound understanding of the medicinal actions of herbs make his books required reading for anyone who is truly interested in herbal medicine.

Michael Tierra

> *The Way of Herbs*
> *Planetary Herbology*

The Way of Herbs is an excellent introduction to herbal medicine. *Planetary Herbology* is a fascinating, eclectic book incorporating points of view from Ayurvedic Medicine, Traditional Chinese Medicine and Western Herbology.

Susun Weed

> *Breast Cancer? Breast Health!*
> *The Wise Woman Way*
>
> *Wise Woman Herbal-Healing Wise*
>
> *Wise Woman Herbal for the Childbearing Years*
>
> *Wise Woman Herbal for the Menopausal Years*

Susun's writings express strong opinions and her books are directed toward empowering women to become involved in their own health care. I highly respect her work and suggest her books to all those interested in expanding their herbal horizons. Susun's poetic side is evident in her work.

Additional reading for the serious student and the health professional:

Bensky and Gamble

> *Chinese Herbal Medicine*

This is probably the most complete herbal book on the use of Chinese herbs.

Finley Ellingwood

> *American Materia Medica, Therapeutics*
> *and Pharmacognosy*

Although first published in 1898, the information in this book is still relevant.

Harvey Felter

> *The Eclectic Materia Medica, Pharmacology*
> *and Therapeutics*

Although first published in 1922, the information in this book is also still relevant.

Rudolf Weiss

> *Herbal Medicine*

This book is an excellent source of modern, useful, accurate information presented in a medical framework.

Notes

Echinacea purpurea

Notes

Passion flower

125

Notes

Arnica

126